T0260520

The Five Health Frontiers

The Five
Health Frontiers

A New Radical Blueprint

Christopher Thomas

PLUTO PRESS

First published 2022 by Pluto Press
New Wing, Somerset House, Strand, London WC2R 1LA

www.plutobooks.com

British Library Cataloguing in Publication Data
A catalogue record for this book is available from the British Library

ISBN   978 0 7453 4393 8   Hardback
ISBN   978 0 7453 4392 1   Paperback
ISBN   978 0 7453 4395 2   PDF
ISBN   978 0 7453 4394 5   EPUB

Typeset by Stanford DTP Services, Northampton, England

Printed and bound by CPI Group (UK) Ltd, Croydon, CR0 4YY

Contents

'Salus Populi Suprema Lex Esto'
The health of the people should be the supreme law
Marcus Tullius Cicero

To Alex

Abbreviations

A&E	Accident and Emergency
ADASS	Association of Directors of Adult Social Services
CSR	Corporate Social Responsibility
CQC	Care Quality Commission
DHSC	Department of Health and Social Care
DWP	Department for Work and Pensions
GHSI	Global Health Security Index
GND	Green New Deal
GNP	Gross National Product
IEA	Institute of Economic Affairs
IPPR	Institute for Public Policy Research
MHCLG	Ministry of Housing, Communities and Local Government
NCS	National Care Service
NEF	New Economics Foundation
NHS	National Health Service
NICE	The National Institute for Health and Care Excellence
NILSS	National Independent Living Support Service
NPM	New Public Management
OECD	The Organisation for Economic Co-operation and Development
OFG	Office for Future Generations
ONS	Office for National Statistics
PFI	Private Finance Initiative(s)
PHE	Public Health England
PHND	Public Health New Deal
PHN-ZERO	Public Health Net Zero
SAGE	Scientific Advisory Group on Emergencies
SDIL	Soft Drinks Industry Levy
TB	Tuberculosis
TUC	Trade Unions Congress
UTB	Universalise the Best

List of Tables

Acknowledgements

It's not always easy to write a book about health during a health crisis. Combining a day job researching health and care with evenings and weekends spent thinking and writing about the implications of the pandemic could at times be oppressive. There were moments I wanted nothing more than to stop, hide away and think about anything else. But this has been a universal experience for many of us over the last 15 months, each witness to the deadly nature of the pandemic and the personal cost of failures in government policy.

In other moments, I felt incredibly privileged. Privileged to have had the opportunity to channel my fear and frustration into the catharsis of imagining what radical change must now follow – and might just become possible. There are few better coping mechanisms.

I could not be more grateful to Pluto Press for publishing this book. Neda Tehrani was an immediate champion for my book from the proposal. She has pushed it in ambition, scope and relevance ever since, for which I'm hugely grateful. Others have made huge contributions throughout the writing process. I appreciate the feedback given by my parents, by Harry Quilter-Pinner at the IPPR on an early draft, and from many others who read chapters or who listened to me read it out loud.

This book would not have been possible without the immense work from the academic and policy community. I am lucky to be able to draw from such a large base of fascinating research and scholarship – it's a book built on the shoulders of giants. I hope what follows does some justice in translating our fantastic evidence into big policy ideas.

Most of all, though, my thanks to Alex – who has managed to be my partner while I dedicated weekends, evenings and early mornings to writing this book over the last 18 months. There is an irony that the health consequences of stress, overwork and burnout are covered in some detail – but she helped ensure I got through all these experiences safe and sound. Sometimes there has been joy, and sometimes it has been a dark and frustrating process. For being there and sharing in both, thank you.

Preface

The idea for this book came well before Covid-19. For a few years, I'd had a half-written book proposal saved in an out-the-way part of my computer. It emerged from my growing sense that there was something deeply wrong with how our public health system works – a fundamental discordance between health today and the democratic socialist ideals upon which the National Health Service (NHS) was founded in 1948.

Often, we chalk 'health' up in the left-wing win column. We talk lovingly about the UK's system of universal care, based on need rather than identity, income, or ability to pay. But the brutal reality is that our public health system still distributes the best health to the people with the most money or power, and the worst health to the poorest and most marginalised.

Today, the most disadvantaged people in our country struggle most to access the healthcare that they need, and experience substantially worse outcomes when it comes to both length and quality of life. These injustices were not eradicated by the advent of the NHS – and they have been observed both in periods in which the health service has had plenty, and in periods where it has been starved of funding.

When news first broke of a new infectious disease spreading across the world, in the first days of 2020, I remember feeling confident we'd be okay. The UK was in an incredibly privileged position. We're an advanced economy, we're an island, we had a well-regarded infectious disease surveillance system, we have universal healthcare, people aren't denied tests, vaccines, or treatments as a rule, and we have an influential role in the global health system.[1]

It quickly became clear that any such confidence was misplaced. To the horror of most in the health, medical and scientific communities – as well as the public – almost everything that could go wrong, did go wrong. Communication was poor and action was often lagging. In March 2020, large sporting and music events carried on, even as infection rates climbed. Lockdowns were repeatedly implemented too late. 'Test and Trace' was established, cancelled, re-announced and then outsourced to disastrous consequence and cost. All the while, tens of thousands of people died.

In an article on *The Plague*, Jacqueline Rose describes Albert Camus' presentation of 'the pestilence' as both 'blight and revelation'.[2] My revelation from this pestilence was that, while exasperated by bad policy decisions during the pandemic itself, many of the problems we faced weren't new. Rather, Covid-19 exposed and exploited structural problems that already existed, only now at a huge scale. In many cases, those structural problems were the same as the ones I had written of in my half-written book proposal.

In some parts, this book tells a story of the discrepancy between the NHS as it exists today, and the intentions and principles set out by Nye Bevan when he founded the service in the late 1940s. But it is quite a different story to the one told in the health books that have come before it. Often, interventions that cover the health service only take aim at the failures of neoliberals, libertarians, conservatives and right-wingers – usually, by sounding the alarm about privatisation. By contrast, this book is just as interested in taking a critical look at the left's strategies to 'save' our NHS. Specifically, it asks why the stories we tell – and the perennial rear-guard action we employ to defend against the wrecking ball of privatisation – are no longer proving either effective or sustainable.

And while it would be difficult to write a book on health without talking about the NHS, I am of the strong opinion that this book is most important when it doesn't talk about the health service at all. Our love of the NHS – 'the closest thing the English people have to a religion', to quote Nigel Lawson – has led to what I call an 'NHS-centrism' on the left. 'NHS' and health have become nearly synonymous among the public, politicians, journalists and activists. But if our goal is to advance health improvement and address health justice, this is far from optimal.

Though it's not a recent finding, it still surprises people I talk to just how much of our health is defined outside of brick-and-mortar hospitals and Accident and Emergency (A&E) departments. Just 10 to 20 per cent of the disparities between people's health outcomes are explained by differential access to healthcare. The other 80 to 90 per cent are explained by factors like our environment, our socio-economic status, or the places that we live in – that is, by our material conditions. This brings into scope agendas and policy levers far beyond the NHS or the Department of Health and Social Care.

To really get to grips with the big questions in health – why life expectancy is stalling, why health inequality is widening, why pandemics are breaking out, why the global health system is increasingly vulnerable and why policy doesn't seem to be making a blind bit of difference – the left needs to expand the passion we have for our universal health service to the other key pillars of the public health system. We need to look at how we've failed to inoculate people against the health consequences of social injustice, and the way poverty expresses itself on our bodies as ill health. We need to look at how we have allowed businesses to profit at the expense of our health, without penalty or shame. We need to look at how a nationalistic approach to health placed us at risk of major health shocks and how it continues to do so. Each of these points is covered by a chapter in this book.

In some cases, the book adds value by highlighting new evidence on key aspects of health improvement or health justice. But, while I have aimed to give attention to drivers of poor and unequal health that traditionally receive less attention, I realise that the evidence on the drivers of poor health is very well established elsewhere, too. This book owes a clear debt to the writers on health inequalities that have come before: Kate Pickett, Richard Wilkinson, Michael Marmot, Lee Humber, David Stuckler, Sanjay Basu, Danny Dorling and others. There are perhaps, then, two places where this book adds value in places less well covered by other works. First, it applies a distinctly radical framing. A key objective here is to bring public health within the scope of the left's wider search for a cogent, coherent and compelling political project that is built around justice.[3] Too often, I find, the health sector and the progressive sector have very separate conversations, using disparate languages – and this book helps to bridge the gap between the two in a post-pandemic moment when our ambitions are broadly aligned.

Second, this book recognises that for all our evidence there is a poverty of radical, left-wing policy thinking in health. The sad truth is that there hasn't really been an exciting health policy since the 1948 National Health Service Act and – for pockets of promising work – health has not hosted the same levels of creativity and ambition as agendas like economic, climate and criminal justice. Now more than ever, we desperately need exciting ideas that explain why public health is important, and why it can be a keystone in a compelling vision of a better future.

In line with that ambition, this book adopts the broadest possible definition of 'public health'. For some, public health means a limited array of local and community services, funded out by a small ring-fenced grant. But in this book, it refers to everything that contributes both to the aggregate health of the population and the way that stock of health is shared out. Public health in this book is therefore not a single arm of the welfare state, but rather a comprehensive and distributive system (akin to the economy). Defined in this way, public health can provide an anchor for a holistic vision for our society and economy – perhaps even an alternative to GDP more suited to the left's goals and agenda.

In thinking about how the left achieve change, I often refer to progressive, left or otherwise grassroot social movements. A key reason for writing this book is to undertake a constructive exploration of the state of the thinking, politics and campaigning around health on the left. Given that, I want to be clear from the outset: I realise the progressive movement is creative, diverse and often in productive disagreement with itself. I therefore realise that when I talk about the 'mainstream', it might lead me to overstate the homogeneity – and that for any critique I put forward, there will be grassroot exceptions. I've aimed to counterbalance this by pointing out a selection of the great examples of activism that do exist in the grassroots. But my main interest is with the mainstream: which left health arguments and topics receive the most bandwidth, the most attention, the most voluntary time and the most funding. Far from erasing the places that are good, my hope is this contribution strengthens the best of the vital work going on in the grassroots.

Another phrase I use regularly throughout the book is 'health justice' – a lesser heard term within the health sector today. More often, we use the language of 'health inequality', 'inequity', or 'the social determinants of health'. We could get lost in semantics here, and I have seen whole programmes of what could have been worthwhile work derailed by an inability to pick a term. I've chosen health justice as it feels better aligned to one of my core propositions: that when it comes to health, we need to be more interested in how power operates, and more cognisant of how we align to other movements focused on radical change and societal justice.

The overwhelming message is one of optimism. I believe that through collaboration, the destruction wreaked by Covid can be the ashes from which the phoenix of better health rises. While we cannot dodge the brutal reality of fundamental problems with the health status quo, this book seeks to provide a new, radical blueprint – one through which public health and care can provide the foundation for a fairer society for all.

Introduction

In February 1928, George Orwell – or Eric Blair as he was then still known – arrived in Paris. He was not alone in yielding to the allures of the city of lights. It was then home to a number of his literary contemporaries – Gertrude Stein, T.S. Eliot, Jean Rhys, Ernest Hemingway and Ezra Pound all among them.

For many, the draw of Paris was the hedonistic 'café culture' of the inter-war period – an appropriate environment for the cultivation of literary bohemianism and high-minded modernist prose. This was not to be Orwell's experience. Instead, his stay in the city would be defined by the shock of a sudden and severe illness.

This experience of ill health would stay with Orwell throughout his life. In the immediate aftermath, the experience informed the semi-fictional *Down and Out in Paris and London* (1933).[1] Twenty years later, he returned to the period, this time in the non-fiction essay *How the Poor Die* (1946). The latter stands as a definitive, blow-by-blow account of the treatment he received during his two-week spell at L'Hôpital Cochin.[2]

HOW THE POOR DIE

L'Hôpital Cochin offered Orwell nothing short of torture. Upon arrival, he was met with an aggressive and unpleasant interrogation by the hospital's receptionist – lasting a full twenty minutes and which, given his feverish temperature of 'around about' 103 degrees Fahrenheit,[3] tested his ability to stay conscious.[4] Next, Orwell was given a hot bath: 'a compulsory routine for all newcomers, apparently, just as in prison or the workhouse'.[5]

His clothes were stowed and replaced with the hospital's uniform of a linen nightshirt and blue dressing gown. In this scanty clothing, he was led barefoot through the open air – on a brisk February evening, and with suspected pneumonia – to the main hospital building. Inside, dim light illuminated rows of beds, each just a few inches, and a 'foul smell, faecal and yet sweetish' filled his nose.

Orwell was humiliated, disgusted and frightened on the ward. The experience led him to conclude that there is a substantial difference between how the poor and the rich die:

> In the public wards of a hospital you see horrors that you don't seem to meet with among people who manage to die in their own homes, as though certain diseases only attack people at the lower income levels.[6]

The most affluent of Orwell's contemporaries could expect to expire in relative comfort. Most of them would pay for a doctor to deliver care in their own home. If they did need to visit hospital, they would book a private room – with better care, nicer food, more focused attention, in short: more dignity. The poor could expect a far more brutal, undignified and painful experience in tightly packed wards. The institution of the hospital, for them, was of the same genre as the prison block or the torture chamber.

Orwell's story is not just about France. It's not pure travel writing, nor is it designed to simply make his British readers grateful for what they have by comparison. Rather, it's a story that epitomises the growing demands in the 1940s for major improvements to the country's health system, and which captures the growing public distaste for the health inequalities present in mid-twentieth century Britain.[7]

It was within this context that the country elected the radical Attlee government, promising a system of universal healthcare. After a long and contested legislative process, the National Health Service was born on 5 July 1948 – with the explicit objective of providing everyone with the healthcare they needed: regardless of class status, income, religion, home address, or place of birth. It was meant, once and for all, to solve the kind of injustices about which Orwell had written.

THE GREAT EQUALISER

The sheer existence of the NHS gives rise to a pervasive idea today that we are all equal in the face of disease. This was certainly an idea that commentators looked to push in the early stages of Covid-19.

The Sunday Express published an official leader to this effect on March 15 2020.[8] In the same month, John Harris wrote in the *Guardian* that 'Coronavirus means we really are, finally, all in this together'.[9] In between the two, the *Evening Standard* declared that 'London Stands Together'.[10]

Madonna, broadcasting from a marble bathtub sprinkled with rose petals, recorded a video message calling the virus 'the great equaliser'.[11]

The actual experience of Covid couldn't be in starker contrast to these early proclamations. The disparities became clear from the moment we first learned the identities of the people dying from the disease. The national media took particular interest in the fate of NHS workers. And as they began to contract the virus, and tragically began to die, it was not uncommon to see their faces lined up on the front pages of the morning papers. Displayed in this way, something became clear: very few of the faces were white.

On 2 June 2020, anecdote was backed by evidence when Public Health England (PHE) published data on the pandemic's inequalities.[12] Compared to previous years, excess deaths among white men had doubled. But among Asian men, they had tripled. And among Black men, they had quadrupled.[13] The report found similar patterns of mortality by ethnicity among women as well.

The same PHE report also implicated class in Covid's injustices, and subsequent data has revealed this relationship yet more clearly. Official statistics now show the occupations with the highest Covid-19 mortality rates in 2020 were, in descending order: bakers, publicans, butchers, police officers, vehicle valets and cleaners, restaurant managers, hairdressers, care workers and home carers, metal working machine operatives, bank clerks, food and drink process operatives, chefs, taxi drivers and chauffeurs, security guards, roofers, waiters, ambulance staff, nursing assistants, catering and bar managers, hospital porters, caterers, and nurses.[14] Every occupation on this list had a Covid mortality rate at least double the average (and as much as twenty times larger).[15] And the clear pattern is that these most vulnerable professional groups predominantly fill jobs that are low paid and unable to offer work from home, but which are vital to maintaining the country.

'Long Covid' – a particularly serious form of the virus, with as many as 200 symptoms according to researchers at University College London[16] – has a similar epidemiology. According to estimates from the Office for National Statistics (ONS), about a million people in the UK had long Covid as of July 2021.[17] Of that million, health and care workers, people aged 35 to 69, women and those with a disability made up a disproportionate number of cases.[18] Moreover, people living in the most deprived parts of the country – a measure obviously related to class and occupation – were also more likely to report having long Covid at the time of the analysis.

So strong is the link between job, class and long Covid, that there have been calls for the illness to be categorised as an 'occupational disease' – to ensure sufferers are eligible for Industrial Injuries Disablement Benefit (IIDB) payments.[19] Despite this, there has been little in terms of recognition, support, or compensation.

INJUSTICE AT SCALE

Severe health disparities are not unique to the pandemic. In fact, the inequalities observed run along the same lines as health injustice before it. Recent estimates put life expectancy for men in the most deprived parts of the country at nearly ten years less than those in the least deprived. Among women, the gap is 7.6 years. The inequality in healthy life expectancy[20] was twice as high – 19.0 years for men and 19.3 years for women.[21] Compared to people in the least deprived parts of the country, those living in the most deprived communities are two times more likely to be diagnosed with lung cancer, and 1.5 times more likely to be diagnosed with prostate cancer.[22] Similar figures can be found for almost every major physical and mental health condition.

That means that while Covid-19 was defined by inequality, and enacted injustice at massive scale, it was not the pandemic that put the conditions in place for this injustice. Covid simply exposed and exploited the existing structural vulnerabilities in the country's health system. The conclusion we must level with is that despite the landmark democratic socialist achievement of a National Health Service in 1948 – and the work done since to solidify and protect those gains – we still have a public health system that disproportionately distributes good health to the wealthy and the powerful, and poor health to the poorest and most marginalised.

It is the same status quo that Orwell and others were railing against, and which was seen to justify radical change, over seven decades ago.

*   *   *

Injustice wasn't the only metric through which the Covid pandemic exposed that something isn't quite right with our public health system's status quo. The UK's overall pandemic outcomes also testify to that fact.

In February 2021, as our vaccine programme began to pick up pace, the UK had experienced 1 in every 25 Covid deaths globally, despite being home to just 1 in every 100 people alive on Earth.[23] Even then, the Covid death count was only suppressed by the withdrawal of universal care elsewhere in the health system. Millions of appointments were cancelled, from routine operations to cancer treatments.

Research published in the spring of 2021 by the Institute for Public Policy Research (IPPR) showed both the extent of this disruption, and the consequences it could have on healthcare in years to come. England lost a decade of progress on cardiovascular disease outcomes, thanks to 5,500 'excess' deaths in 2020. It can expect a further 12,000 cases of heart and attack and stroke over the next five years because of the pandemic.[24] As much as a decade of progress on five-year cancer survival was lost, too, with thousands of extra deaths from cancer now expected from disruptions to screening, referrals and treatment.[25] Elsewhere, checks on people with the most severe mental illnesses fell a third below their target level. Eating disorder referrals amongst children doubled, while treatment waiting lists reached new, five-year highs in 2020/1.[26] Overall, and at the time of writing, the pandemic is expected to create an extra 1.8 million mental health referrals, piling pressure on an already stretched part of the system.[27]

The blame doesn't lie with the individual people of this country. News pages have been filled by pictures of panic buying, empty shelves, packed tube carriages and overflowing beaches. But harder evidence often tells a different story – a British people who were often remarkable for their pandemic solidarity. Most did stay home. The *University College London Covid-19 Social Study*, which followed 70,000 participants over a sustained period, found consistently high compliance with Covid-19 rules – including levels of up to 90 per cent in December 2020 and 96 per cent in January 2021.[28] Mutual aid groups also sprung up across the country.[29] Solidarity funds were set up to help people get through tough times. People made protective gear for NHS workers and came out to clap on Thursday evenings.

The failure is not about individual responsibility. Rather, it's entirely about flaws with our public health system and institutions. Just as in the 1940s, it is evident that massive disruption and destruction must be followed by radical thinking and a bold vision for change.

CRISIS AND CHANGE

Crisis is perhaps the key enabler of change. In the *Communist Manifesto*, Karl Marx and Fredrich Engels describe how:

> a society that has conjured up such gigantic means of production and of exchange is like the sorcerer who is no longer able to control the powers of the nether world whom he has called up by his spells.[30]

Here, the authors refer to a predilection to crisis innate in capitalism. It is an observation often paraphrased as the 'boom and bust cycle' today – a flaw which no capitalist economy has ever been able to resolve. Their final argument is that production will push capitalism into ever greater crises – any one of which could lead to its ultimate destruction.

Milton Friedman agrees on the political significance of crises:

> Only a crisis – actual or perceived – produces real change. When that crisis occurs, the actions that are taken depend on the ideas that are lying around. That, I believe, is our basic function: to develop alternatives to existing policies, to keep them alive and available until the politically impossible becomes politically inevitable.[31]

For Friedman, a crisis makes change possible, but the definition of that change will depend on who wins the subsequent battle of ideas. Elsewhere, various writers, politicians and policy thinkers – William Beveridge, Barack Obama, John Kingdon, Winston Churchill and Rosa Luxemburg among them – have subscribed to the idea of crisis as an engine of radical change.

As crises go, the pandemic is evidently big enough to lead to fundamental change. Covid has had the economic impact of a credit crunch, the human impact of a world war and the societal impact of an industrial revolution. As of March 2021, in the UK, it had killed 125,000 people,[32] caused GDP to decline by 10 per cent[33] and closed schools and workplaces, forcing many to go more than a year without seeing their loved ones. Its magnitude cannot be overstated.

The question is who is best prepared to steer the direction of change when it comes. The thinkers I've referenced, who see crisis as a vehicle for change, subscribe to very different politics. That means the change springing forth from Covid will not be uncontested. Instead, it will come down to a competition of different viewpoints from across the political spectrum – with each looking to define the form our society will take in the aftermath of this epoch-defining event.

We only need to look at 2008 and the aftermath of the global financial crash to see that this is true. As much as the left were emboldened in the subsequent decade, often in bolder and decentralised activism and campaigns, so too were the right. Many countries experienced a significant shift to the right, including dangerous and ongoing lurches towards fascism.[34] Jobbik entered government in Hungary, as did the Lega Nord in Italy. Austria's Freedom Party, Switzerland's People's Party, Denmark's People's Party, Belgium's New Flemish Alliance, Poland's PiS (Law and Justice) and France's National Front[35] are all populist or far-right parties that recorded vote shares of 20 per cent or more at a national election within the last decade.

This is not unique to the financial crash. A 2016 study showed that political polarisation regularly follows crises of this type and severity.[36] In terms of pandemics, analysis has linked major infectious disease episodes to shifts to right-wing populism – including links between Spanish Flu mortality and support for the Nazi party in Germany[37] – but also to revolutions by workers and other marginalised groups: the peasant revolt (fourteenth century England),[38] the 1830 and 1848 uprisings (France),[39] and the riots in Russia that pre-empted and supported the Russian Revolution.[40]

The change coming out of Covid could be radical and just. It could create a better public health system, that distributes good health, more justly, to the people who need it. But we must also take seriously the threat that it could be regressive, or simply magnify the problems that exist within the current status quo. We stand then at a crossroads: in need of ideas, strategy and momentum.

CAN THE LEFT WIN?

Contemporary health movements and activism have remarkable energy. In 2018, I joined a march to Downing Street called 'March for the NHS'. The atmosphere was electric. Tens of thousands of people had taken to the streets, to journey through central London and demand better health. The calls were simple: more money in the NHS, better treatment for health workers and – most of all – private providers kicked out from the system. The march was a demonstration of the sheer passion and energy health inspires. Hours before the set start time, there were impromptu platforms with speakers addressing small crowds of activists. 'Whose NHS? Our NHS!', rang out through the crowd.

There is a reason that health inspires passion on a scale few other agendas do. People care about it for its own sake, and as a site of wider social justice. It is seen as integral to the society we've built, a canary in the coal mine for fairness in our country. The idea of people dying because they didn't have the means to pay for treatment is one of the most abhorrent to our collective imagination.

I admire this. It's one of the reasons I work in health. Nonetheless, there are grounds for stepping back to take a constructive look at the strategy through which the left's movement – the thinkers, politicians, researchers, campaigners, journalists, commentators, filmmakers, social media activists and diversity of people who subscribe to its values – approach the agenda.

There is one analogy that particularly helps us to understand its general nature. The aggregate approach to health in the left movement is reminiscent of how Troy approached its city defences. The NHS has become *the* citadel of democratic socialism, built in 1948 and standing ever since. The left's role has become defined explicitly by strengthening those defences and fortifying the perimeter, in anticipation of ideological assault. We are stuck in a rear-guard action.

That is to say, when it comes to health, our movements, politicians, journalists, thinkers and activists often embody what I define as a fundamentally defensive approach. In simple terms, the logic works as follows. We believe in 1948 as an ultimate victory for the left on the health agenda. The National Health Service, formed by Bevan, is proof that democratic socialist principles can work and that they do make people's lives better. The leftist strategy in health has therefore become defined by maintaining the status quo. If the NHS is democratic socialism in action, then our mission is to protect that from annihilation.

Perhaps it is easiest to define it in terms of what we defend it against. There are a number of perceived threats to 'our NHS': pay cuts, funding cuts and local hospital closures among them. But by far the most oft-cited threat to is the idea of the **sell-off**. Whether in a quick shock-and-awe victory (e.g., an American trade deal) or a more gradual process, the defensive approach is preoccupied with a perpetual threat of the NHS's imminent destruction though some form of mass privatisation. Other issues, from funding cuts to pay-for-service reconfiguration, are often themselves brought back to this primary focal point.

There is, of course, merit in opposing privatisation. Arguments that it is a) not really a risk at all, or that b) it would somehow improve the NHS, are incoherent with the evidence. The former argument has been challenged by the pandemic, which will almost certainly increase the role of the private sector in UK healthcare. As Covid-19 shocked the NHS and stretched its capacity in 2020, the private sector seemed to offer an initial hand of comfort. For example, at the peak of the crisis, independent sector capacity was offered to the NHS at cost price. Yet, we must question the purity of motives when a leaked email from the chief executive of Serco – Rupert Soames – talked of collaboration as little more than a way to 'cement the position of the private sector' in the NHS's supply chain.[41] The message recasts 'generosity' as an attempt to build dependency, with an intention to then exploit.

The latter argument, meanwhile, has been put to bed by systematic review: for example, as published in the *British Medical Journal* by Neena Modi and her colleagues in 2018.[42] Their work shows, first, that private healthcare provision is not efficient: normally, a key argument in its favour. Instead, public hospitals tend to demonstrate either equal or greater efficiency than their private counterparts.[43] Second, they highlight a private sector tendency towards 'cherry picking' their patients – essentially, when allowed to be part of a mixed-economy healthcare model, it scoops up the simplest, richest (i.e. most profitable) patients and leaves the public sector with the most complicated, chronic cases.[44] Finally, they highlight that private companies tend to avoid scrutiny: in the search for a good reputation, few private providers are willing to undertake quite the level of auditing that public bodies undergo.

Despite this, the government has indicated that they are happy to allow the private sector a greater role in the supply chain in the years to come. Rather than provide significant public capacity to get through the post-Covid backlog, the NHS is being forced to procure significant amounts of private capacity. As *the Health Service Journal*, one of the sector's most respected media outlets, discovered in October 2020, private providers have been asked to apply to provide £10bn worth of NHS services over the next four years.[45] This represents a one-off shift to the private sector worth around 0.2 per cent of the annual NHS budget – and though that might not sound like a lot, it is not hard for these kinds of increments to make up a large proportion of the whole.

Even so, a slight increase remains more likely than a wholescale takeover by the private sector. Analysis by the Nuffield Trust indicates there have been two big jumps in the proportion of NHS spend going to the private sector this century. The first was due to New Labour's introduction of independent sector treatment providers and the second came after the market-orientated Health and Social Care Act in 2012.[46] But it is equally true that 70 per cent of the NHS private spend are things that are not often politically contested. The fact that only GPs, dentists and optometrists are in the private sector remains by far the greatest source of privatisation in the NHS and suggests that the left has been broadly successful in preventing further, major sources of privatisation from emerging in the last seven decades.

THE PROBLEM WITH DEFENCE

Evidently there is some danger ahead, but my critique isn't about our opposition to privatisation per se. Rather, it is that the left's movement has focused on defence far too exclusively. In our rear-guard action against the wrecking ball of privatisation, we have arguably forgotten about the other things that matter. And should we find ourselves unable to rectify that, to balance defending what is good about the NHS with a transformative imagination about what a radically better public health system could look like, we will both fail to solve the defining challenges in health today and leave ourselves vulnerable to major problems in the future.

The problem with a rear-guard action is that, by definition, it is interested in protecting the status quo. This leads us to two, critical oversights. The first is an existential threat that could equally destroy the NHS, within decades, should it simply remain in stasis: the spectre of the **buyout**. As much as privatisation and a 'sell-off' would prove destructive, there is equal risk posed by people abandoning the NHS for insurance schemes or direct payment options. If we spend too much time protecting the way things are, and not enough time developing a vision for a genuinely brilliant NHS, we will allow this to happen without adequate scrutiny or opposition.

The second oversight is the limit on how effective and fair a public health and care system we can achieve while only focusing on the NHS. Good health, just health, sustainable health: all rely on the totality of our public health system, in which the NHS is just one part. But a defensive approach predisposes us to overly focus on the NHS ('NHS-centrism'). If the NHS remains the limit of our health horizons, alongside perhaps some limited local authority-run health services, we will miss the opportunity to put forward a genuinely holistic and transformative vision for what good health really means.

THE BUYOUT

Public ownership was a key founding principle of the NHS. But the biggest threat to the health service today isn't an end to public ownership.[47] It is an all-out assault of the extent of its universality.

Nye Bevan understood that the viability of the NHS relied, first and foremost, on keeping performance at the 'frontier' of what is possible. As such, 'Universalising the Best' was integral to his vision, as he told the House of Commons at the second reading of his NHS Bill:

> [. . .] our intention [is] that we should universalise the best, [so] that we shall promise every citizen in this country the same standard of service.[48]

It is a less well-remembered and less oft-cited phrase today, but it is crucial.

What Bevan recognised was that anything less than the most comprehensive health service provides those who can afford it with an incentive to 'buy-out'. That is, it gives them a reason to supplement or replace their public entitlement to healthcare with private health services and insurance – to skip long waiting lists, access novel treatments, receive better technology and digital tools, become eligible for clinical trials, or even to travel to other countries to receive their treatment.[49] The bigger the gap between what the NHS could provide and what it does provide, the stronger the incentive to buy-out – and the larger the group that is incentivised to do so.

The data shows that this is happening. The number of people using private insurance to avoid waiting times is on the rise. In January 2021, market analysts LaingBuisson released a study showing that the total amount spent on private hospital surgery had reached £1.1 billion in value, according to the latest data.[50] That's a 7.4 per cent increase in the self-paying market. A further edition of the research, released in April 2021, showed confidence that there would be further growth in the years to come – with the 4.5 million patients waiting for planned NHS care (as of December 2020) a key driver.[51]

This follows 2017 research by Intuition Communications, which found that profit-driven hospital firms were experiencing a 15 to 25 per cent rise in 'self-payers' funding their own care.[52] And in 2020, Compare the Market – the insurance price comparison website – reported a 40 per cent increase in health insurance sales, compared to 2019, as people looked to insulate themselves against the waiting time increases being brought about by Covid-19.[53]

This fits as part of a longer-term shift. In the 1970s, the UK was the country that used general taxation to fund the greatest proportion of its health services.[54] Yet by 1996, the UK was the advanced economy with the fastest growing shift to 'out of pocket' payments. Where this had accounted for just a tiny proportion of total health spend in 1980 – equal to 0.46 per cent of GDP (value of around $2.5 billion), by 1997 it was equivalent to almost 1.3 per cent of UK GDP (value of around $20 billion).[55] After a small relative drop between 2002 and 2006, the use of out-of-pocket payments to fund health continued its rise – reaching nearly 1.8 per cent of GDP in 2020 (value of around $50 billion). Overall, that's a massive increase in healthcare spend coming from individual, private bank accounts over the last four decades.[56]

A crucial difference between the buy-out and the sell-off is that the former does not need the NHS to be sold, or its budget to be cut. It simply needs public health investment to lag behind the sum of growing need and advancing innovation – that is, to remain in stasis. It is a method of transitioning from comprehensive service to a string-bare safety net that requires little to no expenditure of political capital by the right.

The state of dentistry serves as a warning of the risks this kind of long-term trend poses. In Bevan's original conception, dentistry was within the NHS. The use of charges was introduced in 1951[57] (for dentures) and expanded in 1952.[58] Slowly, over time, charges have risen – with a particularly major acceleration in 1992. As a result, a crisis of access has emerged, and the number of people going to the dentist has steadily dropped.[59] In the place of professional dentistry home dentistry returned. Gut-wrenching stories have become common – of people using pliers to extract teeth or people filling their teeth with Polyfilla and other hardware store products.[60] It's a micro-example of what can happen when we acclimatise ourselves to topping-up our care and allowing the NHS to become an ever-more limited safety net – rather than a method through which we collectively buy the best possible healthcare for everyone.

The existential threat would come in the form of weakened electoral support. There has always been strong public consensus against cuts to the NHS – a service that has provided the best for 95 per cent of the population at a lower cost in tax than they would pay in a market-based private model. This popularity contrasts with the fragility of public support for state benefits – particularly cash benefits for the unemployed. Since the British Social Attitudes survey first began in the 1980s, support for higher welfare payments has oscillated significantly – including sustained periods of support for cutting provision, and more recent support for increasing provision.[61] That instability is markedly different to the consistency of support shown for our NHS – support that sustains its existence.

In the end, it might seem like the buy-out and the sell-off aren't that different. They both end with a conditional NHS, run for profit and unfit for purpose. But we should be far more worried about the buy-out, for three key reasons. First, it is stealthier, and far less costly for the right to implement. Second, it is even more brutally unequal. And lastly, it is a route to reversing the humanising achievements of the NHS – and one for which the left is fundamentally unprepared.

We also need to recognise that reacting to the buy-out requires a very different movement. A rear-guard action makes sense if the threat is a 'big bang'-style sale of the NHS, through either a Thatcher-esque denationalisation process or an American trade deal. But defensive approaches are implicitly about maintaining stasis and supporting the status quo, and that just won't work against the sell-off. Instead, we will need to avoid the space between what health and care the state *could* theoretically provide, and what health and care it *does* provide, from growing. That means having a compelling, radical and transformative health vision for the future – which is not something defensive activism can provide. As such, it is critical to the future of our health and our health institutions that we're able to move onto the offensive, and to articulate a conception of universalising the best fit for the twenty-first century.

NHS CENTRISM: LOOKING BEYOND 'OUR NHS'

Even then, a vision that only focuses on the NHS will not be nearly enough to secure and sustain health justice. NHS-centrism is implicit in any conception of 'defending the NHS'. Yet, the biggest emerging heath and care challenges demand that we look beyond our beloved National Health Service.

In the last 75 years, we have seen a fundamental shift in the country's health needs. The transition can be shown by comparing the big causes of mortality in the two periods. In the 1940s, heart disease and strokes killed 4 in 10 people – often suddenly. Tuberculosis still killed 1 in 20. Infant mortality was nearly ten times higher than it is today.[62] Polio and diphtheria remained prevalent. It was a period when coronary heart disease killed 166,000 in Britain – more than twice as many as the circa 60,000 today (despite substantial population growth since then).[63]

The change since has been defined by three main trends. First, there has been the rise in the age of the UK population, from around 5 million people aged 65 and older in 1948, to 12.5 million people aged 65 or older in 2020. This means the average individual now has more ill-health. Second, a significant rise in long-term chronic health conditions – Type II diabetes, asthma, arthritis and some forms of dementia. Third, the fact that many diseases that presented as acute in the 1940s are taking on a more chronic profile. In 1970, someone could expect to live one year from the point of receiving their cancer diagnosis: today they can expect to live up to six years.[64]

If a rise in chronic conditions has defined the change in health needs over the last fifty years, health in the first half of the twenty-first century will be defined by the challenges posed by 'multiple conditions'.[65] Today, around one in four adults have two or more health conditions – equating to around 14.2 million people in England.[66] People with multiple conditions make up 55 per cent of NHS costs for hospital admissions and outpatient visits. And in the most deprived parts of the country, the average age of someone with multiple conditions is 61 – but lower life expectancy means that they can also expect to live with them for 12 to 17 years.[67]

These statistics all feed into one of the greatest health and care challenges we face: the growing gap between how long we can expect to live overall, and how long we can expect to live with a 'reasonable' level of health. While healthy life expectancy has risen in the last century, it has not risen nearly as fast as life expectancy. On average, someone can now expect to live as much as 15 to 20 years of their life in below 'reasonable' quality health.[68] That means we are spending an ever-greater proportion of our lives in poor health – on average, the entirety of our retirement.

Stalling longevity is also a worry. In many parts of the country, life expectancy was stagnant or regressing before the pandemic[69] – in many cases, due to factors over which the NHS has little control. In a major 2020 review, Professor Sir Michael Marmot implicated child poverty, variation in employment, experience of fuel poverty, food poverty and poverty, rising household debt and the rise of poor housing as the key factors.[70] Other research has implicated obesity.[71] And a similar stall or even an emerging reversal in life expectancy in America has been linked to rising 'deaths of despair' – a now well-established rise in death at middle age amongst people without BA degrees, linked to opioids, other drug abuse, alcohol-related diseases and suicide.[72]

The NHS is best placed to deal with exactly none of these trends and future challenges. It is designed only to pick up the pieces.

For the sake of our health today and in the future, we need to radically reimagine what our public health system can look like. The reality of stalling life expectancy, multiple chronic conditions and an ageing population are more than a treatment service, as one arm of the welfare state, can cope with. Instead, they demand we build a health system that prevents illness, promotes health at every turn, that ensures good lives for people living with chronic illnesses or disabilities. That does not mean hospitals become irrelevant, or that the left needs to become anti-NHS. Rather, it will mean we need to extend our ideals outside of the brick-and-mortar NHS – into communities, into social policy, into our economic models.

The pandemic has added urgency to that mission. It was underlying health conditions – a great many of which could have been prevented by pre-emptive social interventions – that drove vulnerability to the virus. It was occupation, sick pay, access to furlough and wealth inequality that defined whether people could bunker down in their rural second homes or had to work as usual through the pandemic. Covid has underscored the need to view public health as a cohesive, distributive system – in which we proactively increase the total stock of health in the country, and then ensure it is distributed fairly.

With all that said, it is worrying that there are many examples where Covid-19 has catalysed a greater and more explicit focus on the NHS, rather than a broader focus on the whole public health system. One indicative example that has gained traction is the 'NHS New Deal'. At the time of writing, the website for the campaign contends:

For more than 70 years the NHS has cared for us. It's there for us when we need it most. But politicians have continually mistreated the NHS. And during the pandemic, it has come close to collapse. Now we have a plan to win a New Deal for the NHS. This will mean proper funding for our NHS. Support for Doctors and Nurses to do their jobs. Putting the health of patients above the interests of big corporations. Tackling inequalities so that all of us get the healthcare we need and deserve. Our NHS needs you. Last year millions of us clapped for key workers and painted rainbows in our windows. Now we need to turn that support into action.[73]

The copy itself is very hard to disagree with. In fact, it's admirable. But it is also typical of the marginalisation of the rest of the public health and care system from the left's health activism. Until these aspects are mainstreamed in the most developed, most well-funded and most visible parts of the movement, it will be very hard to deliver the kind of advances the post-pandemic world needs.

THE FIVE FRONTIERS

This book is about the health frontiers that span out before us. Based on a decade of research, I have mapped out five frontiers where there are the biggest opportunities to drive forward health improvement and health justice. Some of these frontiers are about reinventing existing institutions and services. Others are about expanding the principles from the NHS into bold new agendas.

The frontiers provide the structure of the book, with each the focus of a chapter. They are put forward as a foundation for a more strategic social movement, one more informed by the future realities and challenges of our population's health.

The inclusion of each frontier is guided by this book's twin aims: maximising the stock of the nation's health, and making the distribution of good health more just. As such, each chapter is designed to stand alone – in putting forward evidence, establishing problems and suggesting transformative new ideas. But each chapter is also designed to fit together into a larger vision: a cohesive new blueprint for better health.

Chapter One begins with the **NHS frontier**. The NHS comes first intentionally. It's an opportunity to dive more deeply into the discourses that underpin the left's defensive strategy and look, in more depth, at how this approach works in practice. I ask whether these narratives are serving us, our health and our health service in the best possible way. And I put forward an alternative – based on the concept of addressing the most pressing issues undermining universal care and based on conceptualising Universalise the Best as a focal point of our movement.

Chapter Two looks at the **Social Justice Frontier**. It begins to define what I mean, practically, by distributive public health. I argue that we need an expansion of Bevan's principles from medical to social interventions – through a new Universal Public Health Service. Fundamentally, this chapter argues we need to be as willing to prevent a health need by giving someone a state funded home, as we are to treat a health need by giving someone a state funded course of chemotherapy.

Chapter Three covers the **Economic Frontier**. It argues that health exploitation by profit-driven corporations is rife. Yet, too often, critiques of this reality are limited by a focus on individual businesses and sectors – rather than a genuine understanding of how this is enabled, incentivised, and normalised by our dominant economic model. I outline the case for a Public Health Net Zero – as a tool to fundamentally change the relationship between health and wealth – and to better protect health from the interests of capital

Chapter Four explores the **Care Frontier**. Care is one of the areas where grassroots and left movements have begun, in places, to expand their horizons. However, while there are some very good proposals, we have stopped short of truly transformative thinking. If today's care homes are the modern equivalent of the twentieth century's asylums, then our policies simply make the asylums free – they do not tear them down. We need to use the foundations of consensus to build a vision not only of how social care provision works, but what social care is, does, looks like and prioritises.

Chapter Five finishes with the **Sustainability Frontier**. It would be easy for the pandemic to make our approach to health more insular, more nativist. On the right, this might come from a greater focus on 'security' – a paradigm that is nationalistic and border-focused. Among the left's movement, it might come from an even more narrow focus on the NHS and outsourcing. This is incongruent with the continuing rise in global health vulnerability – and this chapter argues we need to both comprehend the urgency of the wider health context, and to build a vision for how the UK should now react.

The final chapter brings the frontiers together and explores the case for the Public Health New Deal. I consider how well the interventions fit together. I address key questions such as whether we can afford them, at what scale would we deliver them, and whether we can really prevent privatisation without focusing on it as explicitly.

The shock of war and inexcusable levels of health inequality combined to create the conditions for the NHS in 1948. After the shock of Covid, and in the face of huge health uncertainty and injustice today, the time for radical public health policy has come once again.

OUR HEALTH: A RADICAL NEW BLUEPRINT

1. **The NHS**: A new 'Universalise the Best' mission in the NHS, replacing decades of toxic New Public Management (Chapter 1)
2. **Social Justice**: A Universal Public Health Service, meeting health need long before a diagnosis (Chapter 2)
3. **Economy**: A public health net zero target overseen by a new public health unit, to end health exploitation by capital (Chapter 3)
4. **Social Care**: Expansion of National Care Service concept to cover what care is for, not just how care is provided and procured (Chapter 4)
5. **Sustainability**: UK policy that supports global health sustainability and promises future generations a legacy of better health (Chapter 5)

1
The NHS Frontier

It might seem strange, in a book that has just critiqued the NHS-centrism of much contemporary health activism, to begin by considering the NHS. However, as the institution so explicitly central to how the left approaches health, beginning here provides an opportunity to understand our movement a little better.

If our mainstream narrative can be said to have a common thread, it's Romanticism. The stories our movement tells often rest on a common foundation of the idyll, the emotive, the nostalgic. Our version of barricading the NHS is putting it forward in an idealised form – both to highlight what is right about our politics, and to protect the institution from smear and attack. It is the mechanism we have developed, on the left, to protect and conserve the status quo on an agenda where we believe we have won the argument.

Examples of Romanticism are not hard to find within the Labour Party. One illustrative example comes from Nick Thomas-Symonds' book *Nye: The Political Life of Aneurin Bevan:*[1]

> The National Health Service that he created on 5 July 1948 is no mere monument to his success. Rather, it is a living, breathing example of his democratic-socialist principles, applied pragmatically to bring a better life for his fellow citizens. With a budget of over £108 billion, the modern-day NHS is the world's largest publicly funded health service, employing more than 1.7 million people and providing healthcare to over 63 million people in the UK. Such is the scale of Bevan's achievement that the central principle of the NHS, care free at the point of delivery on the basis of need regardless of wealth, is uncontested by any major political party over 60 years after the service's foundation.[2]

Elsewhere, the story juxtaposes Romanticism of the NHS against the reality of an imminent, existential threat. This was the story told in the 2019 Labour Party election manifesto:

The National health Service is one of Labour's proudest achievements. The right to free-at-the-point-of-use healthcare, universal and comprehensive in scope, is socialism in action . . . [But] A decade of Tory health cuts and privatisations has pushed our greatest institution to the brink.[3]

The manifesto text was brought to life on 27 November, 2019, when the then Leader of the Opposition Jeremy Corbyn convened a major press conference to reveal official documents that purported to show the NHS was 'on the table' in any US trade deal.

In fact, the twinned combination of narratives describing the 'NHS as our proudest achievement' and the NHS as at risk of 'imminent destruction' has defined the party's modern election platform. It's a narrative that brings together Blair and Kinnock, Miliband and Corbyn, Harold Wilson and Hugh Gaitskell. Though the Labour Party's vision and leadership in 1997 and 2017 seem almost irreconcilable, both released final press releases with the same headline: '24 hours to [vote Labour and] save the NHS'.[4]

A Romantic discourse is not exclusive to Westminster. At the opening ceremony of the 2012 London Olympics, director Danny Boyle paid homage to the National Health Service. Set to the music of Mike Oldfield, dancers depicted staff and patients – all set within one of the NHS's most famous institutions: The Great Ormond Street Hospital.

The scene showed little of the realities of healthcare. The hospitals were glisteningly clean. The uniforms were crisp and pressed. The nurses and doctors were numerous and well rested. The child patients were jumping, happily, on their beds. But then, the point of the dance wasn't to give a realist account of the reality of illness or healthcare work. It wasn't Orwell's *How the Poor Die*.

Instead, Boyle's portrayal of the NHS is all to do with the health service as a symbol. The NHS functions as a signifier of our country's progressive capability – our capacity for kindness, our solidarity with our fellow people, our compassion for those in need. Team GB later described the scene as: 'Togetherness, compassion, spirit and support. The NHS embodies everything that is great about our society'.[5]

The Romantic and defensive qualities of the performance were not lost on its audience. Broadcaster Steve Richards, writing in *The Independent*, concluded that:

As the NHS was celebrated vividly with bright lights and hundreds of dancing nurses, I was reminded of *Hamlet*, the scene when Hamlet asks the players to act out his father's murder . . . At the opening ceremony, David Cameron must have felt a little like Claudius as he watched Danny Boyle's players: a Prime Minister who seeks to overhaul the NHS . . . watching a jubilant portrayal of the NHS as it is and was.[6]

That is, he argues that the Olympic ceremony juxtaposed its vision of the NHS against the Health Secretary Andrew Lansley's 2012 Health and Social Care Act – a piece of legislation many viewed as a certain route to massive privatisation.[7]

HEROES

The association of NHS and heroism was by no means unheard of before 2020 – but usage of 'hero' in the same breath as 'NHS' exploded as the Covid-19 pandemic took hold in mid-March. It is hard to pin-point an exact origin, or whether it was steered more from the right or the left. Early articles in media associated with both the right and the left used this framing extensively from around 17 March, as hospitals began to feel significant pressure – and a week before the Prime Minister gave the first 'stay at home' order. Equally, Hansard registers record use of the association spontaneously across parties. The earliest adopters in the Commons registers include Jeremy Corbyn, John McDonnell (Labour) and Ian Blackford (SNP).

Early on, the right's discourse was more likely to be defined by war rhetoric – epitomised in early Covid-19 briefings by Boris Johnson and, in the US, Donald Trump.[8] By contrast, heroism in the NHS has gone on to become the dominant aspect of left pandemic discourse – an image evoked regularly, whether in answer to the poor provision of PPE in Spring 2020 or the government's offer of a 1 per cent NHS pay rise in Spring 2021.

In reaction to the latter, trade union GMB's pay justice campaign called on the government to 'give our NHS heroes a proper pay increase'; The Labour Party promised to 'fight for a significant real-terms pay increase for NHS Covid heroes';[9] The Liberal Democrats 'slammed' the offer of 1 per cent pay rise as an 'insult to our NHS heroes';[10] *The Mirror* ran with headlines like 'NHS heroes take to the streets to demand a pay rise from Tory Ministers'.[11]

There is absolutely no doubt that NHS workers have done remarkable work, at huge personal cost, during Covid-19. Neither does it contradict that reality to suggest 'hero' is a classic trope of Romantic discourse – and one that is not entirely unproblematic. As has been pointed out by frontline workers themselves, heroism suggests a certain sense of infallibility – workers who find strength to persevere, despite overwhelming obstacles. But the reality is NHS workers are human: they feel pain, they have flaws, they get things wrong sometimes and they burn-out if they're pushed too hard.[12] 'Hero' sets a standard of exceptionalism that workers themselves have not always found helpful or healthy.

The hero trope is familiar from its use during times of war – particularly, in propaganda designed to encourage young, working-class men to give their lives for their country on foreign fields. It inspired Wilfred Owen's poem *Dulce et Decorum Est*, in 1918:

> If in some smothering dreams, you too could pace
> Behind the wagon that we flung him in,
> And watch the white eyes writhing in his face,
> His hanging face, like a devil's sick of sin;
> [. . .]
> My friend, you would not tell with such high zest
> To children ardent for some desperate glory,
> The old Lie: *Dulce et decorum est*
> *Pro patria mori.*[13]

The Romanticism of heroism, Owen suggests, ignores the horrors and pains of war, and poorly serves the soldiers who fight in them. Similarly, we must ask if the Romantic, defensive approach we're employing is genuinely serving our NHS and the people who run it.

EXPLORING THE EVIDENCE

Since 2009, the polling company YouGov have tracked the British public's perceptions of NHS performance in comparison to its international peers. At the start of the period, only about one in seven respondents thought that the NHS performed less well than other health systems – while one in three thought it was better.[14] By April 2021, after more than a year of Covid – and as newspaper headlines warned of record waiting times and disrupted cancer care – the number of people who thought the

NHS was the world's best had actually increased. Just one in ten people now thought it performed less well than comparators (down six points), while 42 per cent of people thought it was better (up nine points).[15]

On their own, public attitudes don't really tell us much about whether the NHS *is* the world's best health system. The nuances of the French, German, Singaporean or Canadian systems are not common conversations in the nation's pubs, restaurants, or dinner tables – and few of us have a direct basis for such a comparison. What public attitudes data show is not evidence that the NHS *is the best*, only that the public believe it is.

The study most often used to back up this belief comes from the American foundation the Commonwealth Fund. In their 2017 global rankings, the NHS came top against health systems from 11 advanced economies.[16] That enviable position was thanks to excellent scores for care processes, levels of equity, levels of access and administrative efficiency.[17] The NHS did comparatively poorly in just one area: it comes second bottom on healthcare outcomes.[18]

It sounds like a ringing endorsement, until we consider the nature of the statistic more carefully. The Commonwealth Fund's finding is that the NHS is one of the best health systems in the world, based on everything except what happens to the health of the people who use it. It is the equivalent, in sport, of your team doing well on almost every metric – most points scored, number of passes completed, number of meters run, fewest points conceded, best performance ratings. Except, that is, for the fact they come bottom on games won.

Beyond this famous study, a large body of international evidence indicates that the UK health system lags behind.[19] Research from the International Cancer Benchmarking Partnership puts UK cancer outcomes behind comparable health systems. One major paper emerging from the programme and published in *The Lancet* health journal showed that about 5 per cent fewer people survived for five years with breast cancer in the UK than in Sweden; about 10 per cent fewer people survived five years with lung cancer than in Canada; and about 10 per cent fewer people survived ten years with colorectal cancer than in Australia.[20] In sum, before the pandemic, the UK had lower one-year survival rates for stomach, colon, rectal and lung cancer than Australia, Canada, Denmark, Ireland, New Zealand and Norway. A more general study in the *British Medical Journal* showed that the NHS generally performed below average, when looking at as many as 60 different metrics.[21]

International studies on amenable mortality;[22] infant and young person mortality;[23] admission rates of congestive heart failure;[24] and waiting times for knee, cataract and hip replacement all showed similar results.[25]

The political right waste little opportunity in positioning any sign of poor NHS performance in favour of their ideology – and a move to a more explicitly neoliberal or market-based model of healthcare. Covid-19 has provided them with many such opportunities – as per the below from Director of Communications at the Institute for Economic Affairs (IEA), Annabel Denham:

> concerns about the health service's ability to cope with a second wave and a vast backlog of treatments over the course of the winter [strengthen] an already-watertight case for system-level reform of the UK's healthcare system.[26]

The same IEA has since released a full report that linked the leftist nature of the NHS and the country's poor pandemic outcomes.[27] And the IEA are not the only agitators. Among the right's think tanks, the Taxpayers' Alliance can be found making similar arguments.[28] Similar ideas can be found more widely in a range of commentary, opinion pieces, social media feeds, PR work and press releases.[29]

The aggression of these outriders underpins a defensive approach. But, in fact, it's not the only strategy available. The right's critique suggests that the NHS's problems come down to its democratic socialism. But in reality, the NHS never fails because it is too progressive, but rather only ever where it has been artificially constrained by the taint of neo-liberalism. The opportunity open to the left is to be honest about the problems our health service faces, to relate them back to questions of political economy, and to use these as a basis to expand our values and advance our health further.

To do this we need to understand where a neoliberal political economy has snuck into our health system, what its consequences have been and then how, through reiteration and modernisation of Bevan's principles, we beat it back.

NEOLIBERAL INFILTRATION

The left's defence has not been enough to prevent the infiltration of the NHS by neoliberal ideas. These haven't come through overt privatisation, but rather through more subtle reforms. Slowly, the NHS has begun to reflect the right's ideology. In turn, that reform has created a chronic fragility – reducing the NHS to an ever more limited safety net and meeting the conditions for the 'buyout'. As such, if 'the defensive' is inevitably about maintaining the status quo, we need to think carefully about what we're defending.

The story of ideological infiltration begins in the 1980s. It was an era of wider political change in Britain: the writings of Friedrich Hayek were ever more in vogue; Ronald Reagan had made his transition from Hollywood to the White House; and Margaret Thatcher had begun what would be one of the most divisive premierships in modern British history. It was during this period that the NHS began a transition from an organisation based on the politics of Nye Bevan and the Labour Party, to one run in line with the principles of Thatcherite neoliberalism.

In 1983, Margaret Thatcher commissioned Sir Roy Griffiths – then chief executive officer of J. Sainsbury's – to review the country's health system. His subsequent report is famous for its contention that:

> If Florence Nightingale were carrying her lamp through the corridors of the NHS today, she would almost certainly be searching for the people in charge.[30]

In answer, he recommended a new model of governance and management. He proposed a shift from 'consensus management' (i.e., management of the NHS by healthcare professionals) to 'general management'. Even more significantly, Griffiths put forward an idea that the NHS engage in competitive tendering, a concept that would lead to a new internal market.

Griffiths imagined a system of competition overseen by professionals with degrees in management theory rather than healthcare or medicine. As one commentator put it in the *Health Service Journal*, it was a transition based on 'business school philosophies and experience from the private sector'.[31] While the NHS would escape Thatcher's wider programme of denationalisation, its governance would begin to embody the logic and teachings of the private sector. Neoliberalism through reform, rather than through sale.

The 'business school' approach to the NHS was formalised in 1989 in the government white paper *Working for Patients*.[32] The document detailed a restructuring of the NHS around competition. Most significantly, two functions of the state – budget holder and service purchaser – were split. Providers became revenue-dependent, and commissioners held the money, forcing the former to compete for financing by the latter.[33] In 1991, a further step was taken, with the expectation imposed on NHS trusts of raising revenue from their patients – ushering in an era of expensive hospital cafes, car parks, vending machines and pay per view TV. Patients were now customers in a system fragmented around the dogma of fierce competition.

NEW LABOUR'S REFORMS

Tony Blair's Labour government offered some initial hope of a quick reversal of the Thatcher reforms. Certainly, that was the promise of the 1997 Labour manifesto.

Early on, momentum seemed to be building towards such a reversal. A new approach to health inequalities formally reallocated money to places that were being poorly served. NHS funding increased substantially. In an early White Paper, the government struck back against the internal market by outlining plans to focus on 'integration'.[34] Blair signalled he was personally on board with the shift, telling an audience at the Lonsdale Medical Centre in 1997 that: 'the White Paper we are publishing today marks a turning point for the NHS. It replaces the internal market with "integrated care". We will put doctors and nurses in the driving seat.'[35]

Hindsight is 20/20 vision, and it all jars with the final legacy. It's now well documented that Tony Blair grew frustrated with his inability to steer change and drive improvement in what he saw as Bevan's 'monolithic', state-led NHS.[36] He became ever more convinced that only fierce competition – that is, a return to and continuation of the Thatcher project – could deliver the change he wanted. The school of public sector management he turned to, which had also formed the basis for Thatcher's reforms, was New Public Management (NPM) – an approach often condensed into the motto: 'targets and markets'. It was this adage that, in the end, would really define Blair's health vision.

In came the National Service Frameworks – imposing ambitious, comprehensive, long-term and very top-down targets. 'Strategic Health Authorities' were created to oversee delivery by individual providers, with the power to withhold funding when the centre's expectations weren't met. Fundholding was reinvigorated, alongside strict financial budgeting. Competition was reiterated, with new restraints on collaboration – to the point that providers could not help each other out with small loans. Independent Providers were given a stronger foothold, to compete with and drive on the public sector. A new Quality Outcomes Framework constituted a financial lever to drive up the quantity of specific activities. From 1999 onwards, the new Health Secretary Alan Milburn took on a mission to reallocate significant power to the patient: a choose and book service, review systems and a new look NHS website branded 'NHS Choices' all followed.

The logic was simple. Blair concluded that Thatcher's restructuring of the NHS for competition could be combined with ever more extensive targets, linked directly to funding (a public sector equivalent to profit). Trusts could be made further accountable to budgets and revenue (a public sector equivalent to the profit motive). Greater fragmentation would induce greater competition. And stronger patient choice would create winners and losers, and drive competition (a public sector equivalent to supply and demand). It is entirely in line with the 'business school' ideas introduced by Griffiths – and one New Labour were convinced could herald a new era of infinite improvement.

Undeniably, the quality of healthcare provision improved across some significant metrics during Blair's three terms. However, given that he increased NHS funding massively, after several years of stagnation, this is difficult to attribute directly to his theories of reform rather than to the extra money.[37]

In fact, there are reasons to think that these reforms constrained the NHS's potential, rather than releasing it. Moreover, reports from 2007 remind us that Blair did not leave office with a clearly positive legacy. NHS managers were left dissatisfied by the sheer number of targets enforced upon them, with some suggesting they were wrestling with as many as 300 centrally imposed standards. Big ambitions on health inequalities had translated into a nearly negligible impact, and regular stories about postcode lotteries – rife variations in access to care and treatments based on where one happened to live – continued to dominate the media. The stated prioritisation of patient choice seemed to clash with rising public dissatisfaction with how the health service was run. Despite the money invested, healthcare providers faced major debts and deficits in 2007. And the system continued to struggle with the severe fragmentation and problems with collaboration associated with competition policies.[38]

In other cases, there were scandals within the NHS that suggested the private sector's logic had been implemented far too uncritically. In the private sector, it is well established that the pressures of continuous growth and the profit motive can lead to underhand, undesirable, or exploitative practices – to the detriment of both workers and consumers. In the 2000s, there were echoes of this in the NHS. For example, in 2007, Julie Bailey's mother died in Stafford Hospital. The death opened scrutiny on an unjustifiably high mortality rate among patients being treated there, particularly emergency cases. The Francis Inquiry, convened to investigate the hospital, would find hundreds of unnecessary deaths at the hands of systematic neglect – implicating a toxic culture, unsafe staffing, pace-setting techniques and institutional bullying. In short, the pressures of competition as dictated by NPM.[39]

CAMERON'S COALITION GOVERNMENT

Margaret Thatcher had put in place the structures for NPM whilst Tony Blair put in place the tools to operationalise it. David Cameron took a next, critical step.

In many ways, the coalition's brand of austerity was entirely consistent with the principles of NPM – only now, 'with less' was the keystone. That is, the tools of NPM introduced over three decades were relentlessly adapted to drive efficiency savings, control cost and reduce capacity. As Cameron himself phrased it in a 2012 speech to factory workers in Basildon: 'what you call austerity, I call efficiency'.[40]

An early example was the 'Nicholson challenge' – implemented early in the Coalition years.[41] Under the 'challenge', the NHS was charged with finding £20 billion in efficiency savings by 2015. It would commence a trend – with the NHS's Five Year Forward View strategy asking for similar 'efficiency' savings. Today, it is still common to hear the frustration of senior health officials and civil servants as they find their proposals for highly necessary investment accepted by HM Treasury – provided they can be funded through productivity savings, rather than by actual money.

In the end, David Cameron delivered on his manifesto pledge not to cut funding for the NHS. However, the austerity decade oversaw the biggest deceleration in health spending in history. As the Institute for Fiscal Studies have shown, NHS spending grew at an average annual rate of 3.5 per cent between formation and 1979. It grew at 3.3 per cent per year under the Thatcher and Major governments, between 1978/9 and 1996/7. The Blair and Brown governments also oversaw significant health expansion – of 6 per cent per year on average (though they also arguably proved money alone is not enough without strategy). But the rate of spending decreased in the Coalition years to just 1.0 per cent – followed by 1.6 per cent between 2014/15 and 2018/19.[42]

On paper, it doesn't constitute a cut to NHS funding – but rather a subjection of the NHS to the brutal reality of rising population health need and national demand. The rises in funding – particularly during the coalition years – only just outstripped England's population growth of 0.8 per cent. But once all the variables that increase demand on the health service are considered – an aging population, growing population health needs, the requirements of new technologies and treatments, changes in NHS pay – the funding needed just to maintain the NHS comes to 3.3 per cent. That means the coalition and Conservative governments in the 2010s oversaw major and sustained funding cuts in the NHS.

This subjugation of the NHS to demand pressures is a strategy designed to force a system-wide search for all possible efficiencies, for any 'spare' capacity that can be cut, for any spending commitment or pay rise that can be resisted. While Covid means NHS funding rises now look far more respectable than ten years ago, the same strategy can still be observed at work. In September 2021, the Prime Minister and Chancellor of the Exchequer introduced a new Health and Social Care Levy, funded by a rise to National Insurance Contributions. The money raised meant around £15 billion more funding for the NHS over three years than previously planned. But just days before, extensive research jointly undertaken by the NHS' own representative bodies – NHS Confederation and NHS Providers – had put the direct costs of Covid-19 at £10 billion per year, double what had been allocated.[43] It is another example, even in the pandemic, of the NHS being forced to find efficiencies, just to get by. It is a regime entirely consistent with the treatment of the health service under austerity, and one that both suppresses performance in the short-term and undermines resilience to shocks in the long-term.

CHRONIC FRAGILITY AND COVID-19

Covid-19 provides a case study in the consequences of several decades of neoliberal infiltration. It demonstrates how the shift to a NPM model based on 'targets and markets' and 'do more with less' created a chronic fragility that transformed the NHS from Bevan's comprehensive service to a more limited safety net.

The Partnership for Health System Sustainability and Resilience[44] – a global partnership evaluating resilience across different national health systems – has set out a comprehensive set of measures that define the ability of health services to 'continually deliver their key functions' (including during crisis events). These cover:

- The number and location of beds
- The number and organisation of the workforce
- Deployment of innovation – whether in the organisation of the system, available technology, use of digital and AI tools, or the provision of the best treatments for all those who need them
- A comprehensive health budget (both capital and resource)

These metrics are an excellent starting point from which to explore how, in all but name, reform has undermined the NHS's universality.

Beds were an immediate focus when Covid-19 hit in Winter 2020. Two types of hospital bed are particularly important in reacting to a disease like Covid-19: critical care beds, where the sickest patients are cared for, and general hospital beds, which are more common. As a country, we had too few of both.

In January 2020, the month that would become the quiet before the storm, just 700 critical care beds were open and available in England.[45] These were not equally distributed over the country either. The NHS commissioning region with the fewest beds was the South West. For those reading this book from cities like Exeter, Bristol, or Plymouth, you may be frightened to learn that just 51 critical beds were available for the whole of your region when the pandemic began.[46]

Acute beds were also in short supply. Since 2010, about 10,000 hospital beds have been closed in England. In turn, the UK entered Covid with just 2.5 hospital beds available for every 1,000 people, whereas Germany had 8 and South Korea had 12.[47]

But there is a more important metric than total stock when it comes to beds: occupancy rate. It is possible to have a small number of beds, and still provide safe care – for example, if community care infrastructure is extensive. The best evidence is that safe hospitals have at least 15 per cent of their beds free, to ensure that they can deal with demand spikes.[48] It is a level of occupancy we have not been able to maintain, on aggregate, for years.[49] Just before the outbreak, more than four out of five hospitals had occupancy levels above that safe 85 per cent level. Three out of five had occupancies over 90 per cent. And a full one in four had occupancies over 95 per cent. This would have left them with too little capacity to manage demand, and so no choice but to retract universal care, in the face of even a much smaller health shock.[50]

Of course, hospital beds are next to useless without a team of healthcare professionals to staff them. And when the Covid-19 outbreak began, the UK was in the grips of the NHS's worst ever capacity crisis – driven by the fact we have one of the smallest healthcare workforces in the world, given the size of our population. For every 1,000 people living here, we have just eight nurses and three doctors – both below the average in the OECD.[51] For every 100 people over 65, we have just three professionals providing 'long-term care' – compared to 13 in Norway and an OECD average of five.[52] If the UK – a population with relatively high health needs – were to recruit enough workers to break into the top quarter of OECD nations, we would need hundreds of thousands more nurses and tens of thousands more doctors.[53] These are skilled professionals, who take years to train – meaning gaps cannot easily be filled when a crisis strikes. When it comes to workforce, there isn't really an equivalent to opening a field hospital.

The resources those workers then have at their disposal are also comparably poor. Compared to international standards, the UK offers less of the best treatments to patients. Every year, the government compares the UK's uptake of the best medicines with that of other European countries. In 2019, just 20 per cent of the new medicines available elsewhere were available here, despite having been formally approved based on cost effectiveness, safety and efficacy. It is the same story when it comes to health technology. Compared to other countries, the UK has fewer CT scanners and MRI machines – fundamental pieces of technology for diagnostics. In the OECD, the average is 17 MRI machines and 25 CT scanners per million people. The UK had fewer than 10 per million.

It is the fragility implicit in the dogmatic implementation of 'do more with less' in our NHS that Covid-19 has exposed.

CHRONIC FRAGILITY BEFORE COVID

There's an obvious defence here: namely, that Covid was an unprecedented crisis. Yet, in fact, it wasn't just during the pandemic that fragility was evident. As much as it undermined resilience to crisis, it was undermining people's healthcare before the virus struck.

In 2018, a report by the NHS Confederation established the idea of the 'all year-round crisis' in the NHS.[54] The report systematically demonstrated how a growing mismatch between NHS capacity (supply) and national need (demand) was making it ever more difficult for the system to guarantee people timely, personalised, effective care.

In A&E, they showed a 7.3 per cent increase in attendances between Summer 2013/14 and Summer 2017/18. Over the same period, outpatient attendance at general or acute services increased by 10.6 per cent. The number of people with learning disabilities, autism or adult mental health needs had increased 10 per cent between 2015/16 and 2016/17. Evidence pointed to community services 'running at full capacity'. The number of 999 calls increased by 21 per cent. Yet, across these settings, capacity had either decreased or remained stagnant.

The reality is, without disputing the fact the pandemic has caused clear disruption in the health service, lots of problems we face today are entirely in line with pre-pandemic trends. Take cancer. Data from the Global Burden of Disease datasets show years of improvement in both the death rate and the rate of Disability Adjusted Life Years lost to cancer. Then, from around 2012, the progress begins to tail off. By the end of the decade, it is in full reverse. Had the improvements observed between 1990 and 2010 continued through the last decade, 15,000 fewer people would have died from the four most common cancers (lung, prostate, breast and colorectal). And there would have been 300,000 fewer Disability Adjusted Life Years lost to the same conditions.[55] The British Heart Foundation have identified the same trends in heart disease, with Covid disruptions continuing and accentuating a downward trajectory – rather than creating it.[56]

Evidently, Covid-19 has done severe damage, accentuated by our lack of resilience coming into the pandemic. But we must be careful that the exceptional circumstances of a pandemic do not obscure the structural, political, and ideological underpinnings of our current crisis. It is tempting – emerging on both the right and the left – to explain all instances of NHS strain and poor access to health services through the prism of the pandemic. But in many cases, the blame lies with the failed policies of neoliberalism and austerity.

PUT 'UNIVERSALISING THE BEST' BACK IN OUR NHS

A defensive strategy makes it very difficult to think of ways to expand the NHS and its universality, as opposed to focusing on (at best) simply maintaining it. This is reflected in the policy ideas that have gained momentum – including Renationalisation[57] or an NHS Reinstatement Bill[58] – which are too limited or backward looking to found the distinctly left-wing, forward looking vision of the NHS that re-expressing its universality requires.

If what we need is a re-expression of universality, there is no better anchor than Bevan's principle of 'Universalise the Best' (UTB). Importantly, this is not about a nostalgia-led argument for a return to the NHS's 1948 form – when it was organised around meeting acute health conditions, and its budget was just over £437 million (compared to c.£150 billion today). Rather, it is about expanding and modernising NHS universality – by bringing its reach into new spaces, making it resilient to rising demand and ridding it of institutional injustices that exclude vulnerable people. The five shifts we can coalesce around are outlined below and summarised in *Table 1.1*

Table 1.1   Five Shifts to Universalise the Best in the NHS

	New Public Management	*Universalising the Best*
Extent of Universality	Minimum feasible	Maximum possible
Capacity for Universality	Skeleton-crew	Oversupply
Resilience of Universality	Resilience considered inefficient	Resilience considered essential
Approach to Health	NHS as a treatment service	NHS as a wellness service
Access to Universality	Exclusionary	Inclusive

EXTEND UNIVERSALITY

In tandem with cost-constraint, a culture of risk-aversion embedded by the NPM paradigm is key to explaining the discrepancy between provision of the best tools and medicines to all in the UK – and in other health systems.

Risk aversion is clear in the performance metrics it prioritises and the targets it sets: patient safety, waiting times and financial sustainability. These targets are, in and of themselves, not necessarily bad things

– safety, particularly, is obviously important. But they are targets exclusively focused on managing risk, and therefore managing costs, rather than on alternatives like quality improvement.

This dominance of risk management has very real consequences. Analysis has shown that if the UK were able to meet the standards of health set by its international peers in just four areas – stroke, cancer, cardiovascular disease and dementia – it would add £20 billion to the economy per year; save £10 billion for the NHS per year; and, most importantly, save 20,000 lives per year.[59]

There are many studies and reports that ask why the NHS often struggles, more than other healthcare systems, to get the best technology, medicines, tools and care to all its patients. It is a strange state of affairs, given distribution of the best healthcare was such a clear goal behind the NHS's initial creation. Many of these explorations end up displaying a sense of fatalism in their conclusions: they argue the NHS is just too complicated to ever get a grip on scaling or spreading good practices or lacks the appetite for innovation found in the private sector. The experience of Covid-19 makes these conclusions appear highly suspect.

During the pandemic, something changed: things that we'd been talking about spreading across the health service were scaled, often very quickly. Take general practice. There has long been an ambition to move towards digitally enabled general practice. In 2019, 71 per cent of general practice consultations happened face to face. As of April 2020, 71 per cent of consultation took place digitally.[60] While there are still questions to answer, and urgent questions in the case of the impact of digital exclusions, it still stands up as a remarkable pace of change. Before 2020, many would have thought it impossible.

A digital shift in primary care is not the only such instance. Clinicians have identified a whole host of examples that they find valuable, including rapid access to intermediate care and community assessment, joint working protocols with care homes and 'virtual wards' creating hospitals at home.[61] These are evidenced, have been possible for a long time and are demonstrative of how the NHS has been artificially held back from delivering the frontier of what is possible.

I wanted to understand how this happened so quickly during Covid, when such changes had seemed so difficult before. So, in Summer 2020 I interviewed some GPs as part of a wider exploration of how things changed during the pandemic. Across the board, they affirmed three things:

1. The NHS had developed a very clear sense of mission (fight the virus).
2. The government had got rid of all the bureaucracy and hoops that clinicians had previously been asked to jump through before changing how things are done in their practice.
3. They could access a little money to help get things done, whereas before even small budget requests involved strenuous business cases and were likely to be denied.

More specifically, they talked about how all the artificial instruments used to manage risk and money in a system run according to NPM – like onerous business cases, the policing of collaboration, the abolition of clinical networks and consensus decision making, the tight controls on even small amounts of money – had, at least temporarily, disappeared.

This opens an opportunity for a radical change in culture. At the moment, the health service is organised to react – often discordantly – to instances where patient safety is put at risk, or money unnecessarily wasted. But a missed opportunity to use a new tool, prescribe a new medicine, or try a better practice still causes avoidable harm, disease, or death. Put simply, missed opportunities can have the same human cost as safety incidents. Moreover, being better at taking these opportunities and spreading them does not require us to accept undue risk. Rather, it relies on significantly improving how patients and professionals talk about risk, when making shared decisions on care and treatment.

That is, it requires us to be perennially unsatisfied with the NHS remaining in stasis, against a backdrop of stunning scientific advances and rapidly growing population health need.

INCREASE CAPACITY

Universality relies on resources. And in the NHS, the resource that is most precious isn't, surprisingly, money. It's workers. UTB relies on our ability to end a boom and bust cycle that has plagued our health workforce, and our ability to sustain the most ambitious definitions of universality.

'Boom and bust' conjures up an image of sleepless nights for economists, but is equally salient in the NHS. It refers to our predilection for huge workforce shortages. A historical perspective shows the workforce crisis of the 1940s, when the NHS was formed, and needed an immediate uplift in staff. There was another major crisis in the 1960s, when Enoch Powell (of all people) led a globe-trotting international recruitment campaign targeted at international doctors.[62] There was a further crisis in the 1990s and early 2000s, particularly in the nursing profession.[63] And then there was the pre-Covid crisis when shortages and vacancies blighted nearly every category of health profession.[64] If we include Covid as another, distinct crisis, that's five major busts in just over 70 years.

We run into this problem because, consistent with my discussion of NPM, we have an NHS obsessed with 'just enough'. In workforce planning, this translates to the health sector's own version of 'just in time' delivery. The idea of ever producing *more* doctors, nurses, or other healthcare professionals than the NHS needs is intolerable to the political and policy decision makers across the country. They find the idea of a vacancy far more palatable than the idea of investing in the training of a UK health professional who plies their trade outside the NHS or, worse, outside the country.

There is a relatively simple solution – a shift, in the post-pandemic era, to a policy of oversupply. Simply put, that would rest on an independent body estimating the amount and type of healthcare workers we'll need in the future, and the country then training more professionals than the scenario demands.

In some ways, this will be more acceptable in the twenty-first century than it ever was in the twentieth. As compared to the past 100 years, much of the world faces a shortfall in its health and care workforce – as their population increases, their middle classes grow and the average age of their population rises. There is now a global and humanitarian case, as well as a domestic one, for training more healthcare professionals than the NHS needs.

This will mean some very technical discussions about training places, education pathways and workforce composition. But my research has focused on a second, equally important question: how can the NHS be an employer that actually attracts and retains workers?

There is a very clear discrepancy between people's love for the NHS as a care provider, and what people think about the NHS as an employer. Almost eight in ten people think the NHS is crucial to British society and must be maintained. But only half of the same group would recommend a friend or family member consider a career in the NHS.[65]

One of the best places to start is the most obvious – pay. The suppression of pay in the NHS has been a direct and intentional consequence of a decade of hostile government policy. Most notable was the government public sector pay freeze, beginning in 2010. The result of this decision was a large real term pay cut. At the time of writing,[66] my analysis indicates that the average nurse or midwife has lost around 10 per cent of their pay, compared to a decade ago, after accounting for inflation.[67]

Cuts to pay come with very real consequences. Research carried out during the Winter 2020/1 peak of the Covid-19 pandemic showed that 30 per cent of nurses were relying on borrowed money to pay for essentials. Four in ten had skipped meals to feed their families. Two in three were working overtime to pay their bills. Use of food banks was growing ever more common.[68]

Pay justice is important, for recruitment and retention, but it shouldn't be the sum of our ambition. My research with healthcare workers has consistently shown other needs – including housing, childcare provision, flexible working, progression and time for rest. The hours that healthcare professionals work make it very difficult to balance childcare commitments, particularly if working fulltime, or if sharing childcare with a partner also in the health sector. Rising housing costs put secure, affordable accommodation out of the hands of many in the NHS – represented, anecdotally but shockingly, by NHS workers receiving eviction notices at the beginning of the Covid-19 pandemic by landlords who didn't want to run the risk of key workers living in their buildings. Equally indicative of housing insecurity is 2019 research by the New Economics Foundation, which found that two in three homes built on surplus NHS land between 2017 and 2018 would be unaffordable to a nurse on an average salary, and that just 1 in 20 would qualify as genuinely affordable socially rented housing.[69]

What all this indicates is a relatively simple point. People who work for the NHS want their employment to offer them security, fulfilment of their basic needs, flexibility and hope. They want it to be a place they have the chance to reach their career aspirations, where they can balance work with life and where they can benefit from the security of decent pay, a decent home and decent breaks from the workplace. Until the public sector offers workers those basics, it will struggle to attract enough people into roles, and it will struggle to retain the people it does have through their career.

Perhaps most urgent is action on mental health. In 2021, I ran a survey alongside my colleague Dr Parth Patel, to understand the state of burnout after the second Covid-19 peak. The research showed that 65 per cent of workers were physically exhausted, 70 per cent were mentally exhausted, 50 per cent were working understaffed shifts at least once a week, 25 per cent were turning to alcohol or drugs weekly to cope with work-stress and 5 per cent – equivalent to 80,000 workers – were having suicidal thoughts. The workers had a very clear sense of where the blame lay. Nine in ten said it was down to delayed government policy during the pandemic and a late lockdown. Eight in ten said it was because the NHS had been run so hot during austerity. And seven in ten put it down to the country's unacceptable levels of health and social inequality.[70]

Sadly, this is another instance of Covid-19 exposing a trend that already existed. The health and care workforce aren't in crisis just because of a dreadful two years fighting Covid. They are in crisis because that awful 24 months came on the back of a dreadful decade for workers. According to the NHS's official staff survey, the number of workers experiencing illness due to work-related stress had reached 500,000 in 2019 and nearly 600,000 in 2020.[71] It translates into severe mental health consequences. Mind say four in ten GPs experience mental illness.[72] A paper by Dame Clare Gerada, in the *British Journal of General Practice*, demonstrated how medical professionals experience much higher rates of suicide than the wider population[73] – with female doctors at 2.5 to 4 times the risk of other professionals by some estimates.[74] We cannot expect the best care, from a sustainable number of workers, while we ask that NHS workers simply accept severe mental illness as an occupational hazard.

In sum, our workforce undersupply model is built on a vicious cycle. The life the NHS offers its workers isn't good enough to attract enough new people into its various professions. In turn, shortages drive burnout and poor mental health. More people are put off joining, or otherwise leave the sector. And all the while, the Treasury justifies its chronic underinvestment in workers with the phrase 'labour market conditions' – based on the misguided short-termism that wider economic malaise provides an excuse to suppress pay, terms, conditions and wellbeing in the health service, rather than an obligation to lift it up.

EMBED RESILIENCE

Expanding universality means maintaining the capacity to provide everyone with the best care, even during health shocks. A combination of an ageing population and – as Chapter 5 will discuss – global health vulnerability mean we need to be prepared to handle spikes in demand.

It has not always been the case that the NHS was so susceptible to demand shocks. It has been driven and normalised by a ruthless focus on efficiency, over any concept of resilience or sustainability. The kind of extra capacity that protects us when things go wrong has been redefined, in the last four decades, as needless waste.

I have come across some astounding cases of efficiency being justified over resilience, even in the face of evidence. For some, their reaction to the evidence in this chapter is to acknowledge that there are gaps in provision, but to argue that the country at least delivers said healthcare services at a very, very good price. That is, there is a relatively dominant line of argument that sees the data I've outlined here as a success of efficiency and value, rather than a failure of quality and resilience. That's a big problem, and a narrative that must be challenged and changed.

One of the key learnings of Covid-19 will be that this efficiency paradigm doesn't even work on its own terms. Rather, in its short-termism, it represents an approach that inevitably costs more money when all is said and done. This is plain from a macro-perspective. When a disease that preyed on underlying health conditions and health inequality hit, this country had large numbers of people living with avoidable health conditions and severe levels of health inequality. This made the economic consequences of Covid-19 deeper, and demanded more invasive, regressive public health interventions to stem the damage of the virus. Small investments in health in the decades before Covid-19 would have had huge value propositions and return on investment in pre-empting such a health crisis.

There are some tangible case studies, too – perhaps the best of which is the cost of the Nightingale hospitals. The Nightingale fleet was only necessary because of a lack of capacity in the health service. They were required to maintain confidence in the NHS avoiding collapse, because bed numbers, occupancy levels and ICU capacity were all uncertain in Spring 2020. No data embodies this fact better than the fact the Nightingales were hardly used. The London site saw just 54 patients during the pandemic's first wave. Estimates suggest that spending on the Nightingale's will total somewhere between £500 million and £1 billion. Some estimates put the cost at over £1 million per patient in the year 2020, a cost equal to fifty cancer treatments.

Had we embedded a UTB principle before the pandemic, we would have secured the same surge capacity far more proactively. For example, evidence has pointed out a dual problem with hospital discharge in the NHS – namely, some patients being discharged far too quickly (and therefore returning) and others far too late. The combined cost of these two trends is an estimated £3 billion per year.[75] Investing the Nightingale funding into better discharge processes and more community access before the pandemic – rather than waiting until a crisis hit – could have freed up hospital beds, saved money and tangibly helped people. It could, indicatively, have funded a massive rise in community capacity: 50 million hours of community care to support discharge, 20–30 million physiotherapy services or 17 million one-to-one occupation therapy sessions. All of these are excellent ways of improving discharge.

The challenge is finding a simple policy lever through which to embed maintenance resilience as the new common sense in health service management. Any solution will need to ensure straying from resilience costs political capital. In 2020, I proposed one such approach.[76] I suggested that the UK government borrow from economic policy's 'fiscal rules' and introduce 'health and care resilience rules'. In the Treasury, the fiscal rules are designed to embed political accountability around consistent and long-term focused economic policy. In health, these rules could include:

1. *A Capacity Rule*: We should open enough hospital beds to reach safe occupancy levels in hospital.[77] Thereafter, any hospital bed closures should only be allowed if there is pre-emptive and equal investment in other settings (home care, community care, social care).

2. *A Staffing Rule*: A commitment to reach and maintain, at the very least, the average workforce per capita in comparator countries – across medical, nursing, allied health, ambulance and community professions.

3. *A Modernisation Rule*: A commitment to making available at least the same number of National Institute for Health and Care Excellence (NICE) approved and cost effective treatments to England patients as made available in other advanced countries – and to ensure we match other countries on technology, data and digital tools.

4. *A Sustainable Funding Rule*: NHS funding made equal, in the first instance, to the average investment in the G7 (ignoring one-off Covid-19 investments) – with funding used to enable transformation and resilience.

Combined with regular reporting, these rules could help set expectations and ensure political cost when those expectations are breached.

FROM TREATMENT TO WELLNESS

The trajectory of changing population health needs means NHS universality will only be assured when it can provide for the reality of multiple conditions and wide inequalities.

The reality of people being diagnosed with multiple chronic conditions – perhaps arthritis, combined with depression or anxiety, alongside COPD or angina – means changing our model to one that can provide more holistic support. People no longer need just intensive support in hospitals (a treatment service). They need help to cope with chronic conditions, and to still live brilliant lives within their homes and community (a wellness service).

There are emerging examples of services yielding fantastic results by going *to* people in the places they live, making better use of community and charity services,[78] and treating the whole person, not just their illness.

In Glasgow, a programme called 'Improving the Cancer Journey' was launched in 2014. It serves a community support service, providing everyone with an individualised assessment and care to local people diagnosed with cancer. The needs assessment covers not just physical, but emotional, family, practical and spiritual needs – going far beyond ideas and services traditionally seen as within the health service's remit. Its focus on outreach and presence in the place where people actually live – rather than in out of the way, medicalised settings – meant it was incredibly beneficial and accessible for people living in more deprived parts of the city, and those living with more complicated or multiple physical and mental health needs.[79] Elsewhere, 'hub models' – community clinics with GPs, but also local authority, charity, co-operative and voluntary sector services – are having an impressive impact.

The problem is, these kinds of services are currently only possible in isolated instances, and where they have access to voluntary sector funding. They do not represent fundamental changes in the NHS's publicly funded service offer.

Indeed, estimates suggest community care services and infrastructure have actually been significantly cut back in recent years.[80] Changing this trajectory, and extending the NHS beyond hospitals, is critical to Universalising the Best, ensuring equality of access to health services and ensuring universality in the face of changing health challenges in the decades to come.

ELIMINATE INSTITUTIONAL INJUSTICE

An obvious case of institutional injustice in the NHS is the interaction between British colonialism and the origins and evolution of the National Health Service. The NHS's existence was only made possible by the international workforce that staffed it, upon its creation in 1948. Indeed, its existence came in the same year that the passengers of the HMT Empire Windrush landed in the Port of Tilbury. They landed to find a newly formed NHS in desperate need of their labour,[81] and many would go on to staff this ambitious new public service.[82]

Ever since, our NHS has remained viable because of its global workforce. Throughout history, we have answered workforce shortages with massive international recruitment campaigns. Before he spoke of 'Rivers of Blood', Enoch Powell launched and led an overseas campaign to find and recruit trained doctors – bringing in 18,000 new staff from India and Pakistan alone.[83] Today, the UK workforce is more international than almost any other in the world. 15.4 per cent of UK nurses and 29.2 per cent of UK physicians were trained in another country – compared to an average amongst EU 15 countries of 4.2 and 15.1 per cent respectively.[84]

This is often presented as a point of pride. Matt Hancock MP has talked about 'the benefits of a diverse, international workforce' and about 'welcoming even more incredible talent to our health system'.[85] At his 2018 conference speech, the Labour Shadow Minister for Health Jonathan Ashworth gave his thanks to 'those who have come from across the world to care for our sick and elderly whether from the EU, the Indian sub-continent and yes the Windrush generation too'.[86]

By ignoring that this system is built on the back of exploitation, such uncritical pride amounts to rank hypocrisy. Despite its reliance on healthcare professionals trained in Britain's former colonies, the NHS was an integral participant in the formation of the 'hostile environment' pioneered by Theresa May as Home Secretary. For example, new regulations introduced in 2015 require NHS Trusts to charge people who are not eligible for NHS care at 150 per cent of the cost of that care. The same regulations introduced an Immigration Health Surcharge – a fee levied on UK VISA applications, including for NHS workers, on top of other Home Office immigration charges.[87]

The scheme serves a dual purpose within government policy. First, it allows the government to further embed their culture of 'do more with less'. Even though the government's own estimates put the cost of NHS 'misuse' by international visitors at just £300 million, an extensive effort to reclaim these funds communicates the extent to which they'll go to retain money. More importantly, as highlighted by grassroot campaign group Docs not Cops, it helps create an environment of surveillance and overt repression. That is, a legal duty on NHS Trusts to charge is also a legal duty on NHS Trusts to undertake extensive immigration checks, and to employ their privileged access to data in support of the hostile environment. It is even more powerful because it comes through a service that we cannot do without.[88]

Put simply: the NHS only functions because of the contributions of an international workforce – past and present. In many cases, their education and training has been funded abroad, and the extent to which the UK relies on international recruitment often draws workers away from countries where they are also needed. The World Health Organisation estimates that 18 million more health workers are needed to achieve universal healthcare in low and lower-middle income countries by 2030 – a target from which the UK evidently detracts.[89] And yet, those same workers have been deployed as part of a regime designed to police migrants, control borders and enact a hostile environment.

The severe health impacts of the Windrush scandal – whereby hundreds of Commonwealth citizens, many from the 'Windrush' generation, were wrongly deported or denied legal rights – brought this story full circle. The policing of access to the NHS constituted a denial of healthcare for many who had come to the UK as part of the same Windrush generation that filled the NHS immediate labour needs in the 1940s. Of course, the right to healthcare should be a human right for all migrants – regardless of their economic contribution. Nonetheless, juxtaposing the economic contribution demanded of migrant people by the British state, with its reluctance to extend human rights and the welfare state, gives a clear sign of our hypocrisy and of health's continued struggles with colonialism and colonial structures.

Institutional injustice in health is not just about individual scandals. If the NHS is a system tainted by colonialism, then the impact can be seen in how well its services are designed around the needs of people from

Black, Asian, or Minority Ethnic backgrounds. From this perspective, we see a system that translates colonialism into a universally poorer offer for many people today.

Where there is data – and health data on ethnicity is often limited – there are signs of a big problem in how Black patients are treated within the NHS. For example, every year, the NHS releases results of its Cancer Patient Experience Survey – giving a comprehensive overview of what people think about their cancer care. There are sixty questions, all covering different interactions with the health service. Nine of those questions do not have a breakdown for ethnicity. Of the remaining fifty-one questions, my analysis for this book shows that Black people have worse experiences on 40 metrics. People from Asian backgrounds have worse experiences on 46 metrics. Particularly notable disparities include:

- Black and Asian people having to visit their GP more times before they are referred, indicating their symptoms are not taken as seriously
- Black and Asian people more often indicating their test results were not explained in a way they could understand
- Black and Asian people more likely to indicate they were not treated with respect and dignity in hospitals

These are indicative of an NHS that remains structured in a way that is discriminatory, more amenable to the needs of white people and retains the fingerprints of institutionalised, enduring colonialism.[90]

To some extent, this is depressingly unsurprising, given who designs and leads the NHS as a health institute (and has done through its whole history). Despite the introduction of a Workforce Race Equality Standard (WRES) in 2015, problems continue in Black representation, particularly in leadership positions. Across the whole country, 20 per cent of staff in NHS Trusts and Clinical Commissioning Groups are from a Black, Asian or minority ethnic (BME) background. But they represent just 8 per cent of NHS board members.[91] And they are significantly underrepresented in the highest pay bands – with just 6.5 per cent of BME workers in 'very senior management' positions.[92]

This isn't down to a deficit in talent, and there are signs that people from minority ethnic groups have their progress stymied by bosses and colleagues. Research from just last year found that workers from minority ethnic backgrounds were twice as likely to have experienced discrimination or unfair treatment from a colleague or a manager.[93]

Unsurprisingly, a system designed by white British people and managed by white British people provides better access and outcomes for white British people. Recent government research has shown that Black women are both the most likely to develop depression and anxiety disorders, and the least likely to receive mental health treatment for these same disorders.[94] Worse, Black adults are significantly more likely to be sectioned under the Mental Health Act.[95] There are discrepancies outside of mental health, too. For instance, the end-of-life care charity Marie Curie found discrepancies in whether someone has dignified, high quality palliative care – attributable to race – meaning people dying less dignified and more painful deaths for no clinically justifiable reason.[96]

This kind of exclusion is in line with the priorities of the system that has developed over the last four decades. A focus on financial sustainability, one-size-fits-all targets, competition and efficiency actively incentivises healthcare providers to ignore those with more complicated (and expensive) health needs. That is, it encourages them to sustain existing inequality. A left approach based on romanticising the NHS is, equally, poorly optimised to challenge this reality. In approaching health as an agenda we've won – and a status quo to preserve – we lack the natural scepticism of state institutions found in activism against prisons, the police or the Home Office's deportation regime.

Of course, it's important not to erase areas where this problem is focused on by excellent grassroots movements. Decolonising Contraception, MedAct and Black Lives Matter have all done excellent work in pushing these important issues and stories into prominence. A definitive test of our movement will be whether these kinds of experiences and statistics can come to drive the same campaign activity seen around questions of privatisation; or when deaths from poor health attributable to racism cause the same outcry as deaths attributable to racism within the Metropolitan Police.

We need to be able to look honestly at the problems within our NHS, bring that radical critique back to questions of politics and ideology, and push transformative justice. It is a need that conflicts with the desire to defend and romanticise the NHS. It is one of the clearest reasons for an adjustment in our movement's strategy.

2

The Social Justice Frontier

Our ambition cannot end with the National Health Service, no matter how much more expansive. Health improvement and health justice, the twin aims of this book, demand we focus beyond just one institution and look at public health as a whole system.

Just as an economist might be interested in both the total sum of wealth, and how that is then shared out, the coming chapters are interested both in how we can increase our stock of good health and, perhaps more importantly, how we can create a public health system that distributes good health fairly.

This line of enquiry brings us back to Orwell's observation, with which I opened the book: why is that some conditions seem to only (or more aggressively or more regularly) attack people at the lower income levels?

Orwell immediately turns to hospitals and health settings for his own explanation in *How the Poor Die*, a premonition perhaps of contemporary NHS-centrism. But there is another work from the progressive canon that provides an even more accurate explanation of the political economy of public health today.

WHY WAS TINY TIM SICK?

Charles Dickens' *A Christmas Carol* follows the archetypal miser Ebenezer Scrooge, a man who is mean with his money, even to his own detriment, who neither invests in his own comforts, nor entertains philanthropy. Bob Cratchit is the unlucky clerk in Scrooge's employ, and as a result faces a severe combination of low pay, long hours and poor living conditions. His poverty is compounded by circumstance. Bob and wife Emily have four children – the youngest of which, Tiny Tim, is seriously ill. Dickens describes the boy as cheerful and full of spirit, as per his famous line: 'God bless us, everyone'. But his illness is worse than can be solved by a positive disposition. When Scrooge is visited by the Ghost of Christmas Yet to Come, he sees that, should the timeline continue unchanged, Tiny Tim will die.

Dickens does not give Tiny Tim a diagnosis, but many have since taken on the medical detective work. A review by Dr Russell Chesney in *the Archives of Paediatric and Adolescent Medicine* summarises the most likely suggestions: Rickets; Tuberculosis (or a combination of the two); Renal Tubular Acidosis (Type 1);[1] or simple malnutrition.[2] These hypotheses help us understand what Tiny Tim would have needed to survive.

A common thread among all these potential diagnoses is that he would have needed interventions that sit outside the gift of even the modern NHS. Malnutrition is a disease of diet, rickets either of diet or exposure to sunlight. Renal Tubular Acidosis would have demanded exercise, sunlight, better diet, or even a supplement of sodium bicarbonate. Chronic tuberculosis could be prevented, or managed, with increased Vitamin D[3] – particularly, if diagnosed in tandem with rickets.[4]

As the Ghost of Christmas Present shows Ebenezer Scrooge, Tiny Tim's ailment would have been fatal should his poverty have continued. His salvation is not down to a new medical discovery, the creation of a new health service, a lucky improvement in condition, or advancement through individual merit on the part of his father. Rather, the difference between Tiny Tim dying and surviving is the reformation of Ebenezer Scrooge – and the fairer living standards that become available to the whole Cratchit family thereafter. That is, the end of his family's poverty saves his life.

THE TWENTY-FIRST CENTURY TINY TIMS

Two centuries on, *A Christmas Carol* is remarkably in-line with the workings of health distribution and injustice in Britain today. The link between poor health and poverty has not been severed and continues to afflict millions with avoidably worse health.

In fact, we can use Tiny Tim's experience of ill-health to draw a genealogy between the Cratchit's circumstances and millions of 'modern day Tiny Tims'. Rather than give a passing list, I look at two aspects of the Cratchit's poverty in detail: housing and employment.

Dickens describes the cramped quarters the Cratchit's live in, six people sharing four squat, smoke-filled rooms. Like Dickens' childhood home, the Cratchit's house is in London's Camden Town – a place the author would have associated with his own poverty and his father's imprisonment in debtor's prison. Later in life, Dickens described Camden as 'a complete bog of mud and filth with deep-cart ruts, wretched hovels, the doors blocked up with mud'.[5]

Today, housing continues to determine the health of millions. The English Housing Survey shows that 10 per cent of the UK's housing stock has what are known as 'Category 1 Hazards', including a disproportionate 600,000 homes in the private rented sector.[6] Category 1 hazards include serious and immediate dangers. There might be asbestos, a well-known cause of fatal lung conditions. There might also be serious mould or fungal growth – which can cause health problems for all but are particularly dangerous for those living with an existing respiratory condition like asthma. There could be carbon monoxide – the so called 'silent killer' – or other lethal substances, like lead or nitrogen dioxide.

Elsewhere, poor housing creates what are often wrongly seen as small discomforts, which can nevertheless snowball into serious health conditions. Just as Bob struggles for warmth in the opening scenes of Dicken's novella, millions today struggle to heat their homes in the UK. According to recent government data, an estimated 2.4 million households in England live in fuel poverty.[7] People who experience this are likely to try to 'put up' and cope the best they can. They might use their heating intermittently: for an hour a day, otherwise tolerating the cold. They may limit their lives to one or two rooms, which they can afford to heat more often. They may be forced to make a daily choice between heating or eating.[8]

Health consequences follow. One study by the Institute for Health Equity found that cold homes are linked to reduced weight gain in infants, asthma in young children, mental ill-health, increased incidence of flu, worse episodes of arthritis and (amongst old people) increased chance of heart attack, stroke, or chronic lung disease.[9] In any given year, tens of thousands of people die just because of excess cold – an epidemic on a similar scale to Covid, and one that is entirely preventable.[10]

As important as the quality of housing is the level of crowding within. Overcrowding affects 800,000 people today.[11] It is a plight almost exclusively experienced by people renting their homes – with 8 per cent of social renters and 6 per cent of private renters living in overcrowded conditions respectively.[12] From a health perspective, it is a key factor in the prevalence of Tuberculosis (TB) in this country. One study in London showed that when overcrowding increased by 1 per cent, TB infection rates also rose by 1 per cent.[13] Covid-19 was another infectious disease where cramped housing was tindering to rapid spread. Like many comparable diseases, Covid spreads more easily in indoor settings where people are in regular proximity. The government's Scientific Advisory Group for Emergencies (SAGE) not only identified a correlation between crowded houses and Covid-19 mortality but observed that link independently of the wider impacts of socio-economic deprivation.[14]

These figures come on the back of a litany of recent policy failures. In 2004, proposed legislation on a statutory overcrowding standard was touted but not introduced. A 2007 government pilot on overcrowding wasn't scaled. The Coalition government's 2011 Localism Act provided new tools to assess overcrowded housing but was reliant on the proactivity and good will of landlords, leaving renters at the unsympathetic whims of capital. Unsurprisingly, this meant little progress. New provisions on overcrowding proposed in the Lords stages of the 2016 *Housing and Planning Act* were withdrawn. All the while, homes continue to get smaller. The UK average new build is 76 square meters, the smallest in Europe[15] – and unaffordability continues to drive average occupancy of those homes up.

When compiled, one in seven of us live in unaffordable, insecure, or unsuitable homes – according to State of the Nation research by the National Housing Federation.[16] That's 8.4 million people: 3.6 million in overcrowded homes; 2.5 million in homes where they can't afford the mortgage or rent; 2.5 million living with parents or an ex-partner or friends; 1.7 million people in unsuitable housing – for instance, where they have a physical disability and can't get around or out their home; and 400,000 people at risk of homelessness. They have been let down by poor regulation, by a lack of social housing and by a government obsession with artificially inflating house prices. Like Tiny Tim, their access to health – regardless of their access to the NHS – is being sacrificed.

RACIALISED HEALTH INJUSTICE

In *A Christmas Carol*, Dickens does not go beyond poverty. But there is an onus on us to take the analysis further. Then and today, it's not only poverty that defines how health is distributed, it is also circumscribed by structures like race and gender.[17] The case study of work gives a clear insight into how racism, class and poverty interact to define the distribution of public health in modern Britain.

There is rich historic evidence showing how the nature of work impacts health. Beginning in 1967, the 'Whitehall study' of British civil servants looked at whether there was a link between grade of employ-ment and mortality from disease.[18] The study tracked the health of thousands of British officials over a period of years, conclusively demon-strating that those in more junior roles had higher health risks and, in turn, a greater susceptibility to avoidable, premature mortality. Indeed, men in the lowest grades of work a three times higher mortality rate than men in the highest grades of work.

A follow up to the study published in *The Lancet* health journal in 1991 confirmed that there had been no reduction in the link between low-paid work and recommended 'more attention . . . be paid to the social environments, job design and the consequences of income inequality'.[19]

These might seem studies about class, but they are also absolutely studies in race – not least because the injustices of race and class can never be entirely separated. White people are more likely to have access to the well paid, fulfilling jobs that predict better health outcomes. In Whitehall today, ethnic minorities make up just 7–8 per cent of the senior civil service, but 12 per cent of civil servants overall and 11 per cent of the country's population.[20] That means that while Black people are taking up jobs that are essential to the functioning of the country and its public services, they are disproportionately exposed to work-related health risks, which impact both the quality and length of their life.

One of the experiences that best links the Cratchits with tens of thou-sands of Black people and families today is precariousness. Insecurity is a plight to the Cratchit family – Bob has little power in the face of his employer.[21] Today, the same sense of insecurity and lack of recourse is felt in many workplaces – but most of all, in the 'gig economy'.

In 2017, the government published the findings of the Taylor review into modern working practices. The review found that white workers were severely underrepresented in the gig economy. Indeed, just 68 per cent of gig economy workers described themselves as white British.[22] Elsewhere, it has been shown that Black workers are twice as likely to be on zero-hour contracts, as compared to white workers – driven in par-ticular by a rise in Black women on zero-hour contracts, according to the TUC.[23]

Emerging research paints a bleak picture of the health consequences. A 2020 study for the Royal Society of Public Health's journal showed that workers paid on a 'piece rate' – that is pay per delivery made, job com-pleted, or item produced – decreased workers' health, in comparison to salaried workers.[24] Piece rate is a growing tool to push productivity, not only in the gig economy, but in places like Amazon fulfilment factories. While not as obviously a health risk as heavy machinery, it is absolutely a high-impact occupational hazard.

Another study, led by Ursula Huws – professor of labour and globalisation at the Hertfordshire School of Business – identified some of the specific occupational health risks within gig economy roles.[25] These included physical risks – riding a bicycle to deliver food on busy London roads; sitting in a car for long periods;[26] a lack of proper health assessment; using equipment, like hot irons, without formal training.[27] They also included mental health risks – from waiting for work for hours; having to cancel social plans because a last minute shift came through; and feeling unable to say no to work, in case you're deactivated or deprioritised by your employer.[28]

These are all before we even bring in the question of pay. By the government's own figures, one in four in the gig economy earned less than £7.50 per hour in 2018 (the minimum wage that year).[29] Low pay is directly associated with poor health – both mental, including everything from stress to trauma, and physical, from respiratory problems through to heart disease.[30]

This can create a vicious cycle for those affected. One of the key barriers to secure, well-paid work is chronic illness or disability.[31] Poor work and low pay in turn create and sustain the conditions for worse health. It is only too easy to be caught in a cycle of reinforcing health and economic injustice. This is central to the inhumanity behind the Coalition government's austerity era Make Work Pay policies.[32]

While the gig economy comes with specific risks, the link between illness and racism is not just a problem of one sector. It infects the whole economy. Regardless of where they work, Black people are then more liable to experience a whole range of occupational health hazards within the workplace. In 2005, a study commissioned for the Health and Safety Executive concluded that – when looking at white people and people from minority ethnic backgrounds, of similar ages and roles – the latter were far more likely to experience stress and that the reasons for that stress was, explicitly, racial discrimination.[33] Seventeen years later, things haven't changed. The recent McGregor-Smith review documented that workplace disadvantages were still impacting the health of Black, Asian and minority ethnic people.[34]

When Dickens wrote his novella there were some instances of public health improvement underway, perhaps none more so than sanitation works to provide more people with clean water. Today, long working hours, bad bosses, receding workplace rights, poor private sector housing and precariousness are the equivalent of dirty water – killing hundreds of thousands each year, and sustaining disparities along the lines of race, occupation, class and material conditions.

Today's equivalent of the sanitation works would eliminate bad landlords, bad bosses and poverty.

WHY HAS NOTHING CHANGED?

There is clearly value in compiling the latest evidence. But I'm not the first person to highlight these drivers of poor health. In 1980, the *Black Report* was a landmark in establishing structural drivers of health inequality.[35] In 2010, Michael Marmot's report *Fair Society Healthy Lives* established a whole host of 'social determinants of health' beyond what is in the scope of a medical health service.[36]

And while these reports stand out as seminal, even they don't constitute particularly revolutionary additions to overall knowledge. The first national Whitehall department for health – the Ministry of Health, set up in 1919 – contained functions well beyond hospitals. It oversaw National Insurance, the Poor Law, local government, community planning, housing and environmental health.[37] That is, it demonstrated a fundamental understanding – and a far better one than often seen today – of the need for a holistic definition of health.

Political and policy inaction on poverty and health – or racism and health, gender and health, transphobia and health – hasn't been enabled by a paucity in our knowledge. There are two more important reasons that good public health research has not been translated into truly radical policy change. First, the continued dominance of the idea of personal responsibility for our health, which constrains the scope for state-led interventions. Second, a lack of totemic ideas around which advocates of an alternative can coalesce.

We can return to *A Christmas Carol* for illuminating commentary on the idea of personal responsibility. It's the politics of choice for the unreformed Ebenezer Scrooge – one that allows him to justify his miserliness; the hawkishness of his business practices; and the brutality of his employment standards.

"Are there no Prisons?" asked Scrooge.

"Plenty of prisons," said the gentleman, laying down the pen again.

"And the Union workhouses?" demanded Scrooge. "Are they still in operation?"

"They are. Still," returned the gentleman, "I wish I could say they were not."

"The Treadmill and the Poor Law are in full vigour, then?" said Scrooge.

"Both very busy, sir."

"Oh, I was afraid, from what you said at first, that something had occurred to stop them in their useful course," said Scrooge.

"Under the impression that they scarcely furnish Christian cheer of mind or body to the multitude," returned the gentleman, "a few of us are endeavouring to raise a fund to buy the Poor some meat and drink, and means of warmth. We choose this time, because it is a time, of all others, when Want is keenly felt, and Abundance rejoices. What shall I put you down for?"

"Nothing!" Scrooge replied.

"You wish to be anonymous?"

"I wish to be left alone," said Scrooge. "Since you ask me what I wish gentlemen, that is my answer. I don't make merry myself at Christmas, and I can't afford to make idle people merry. I help support the establishments I have mentioned: they cost enough: and those who are badly off must go there."

"Many can't go there; and many would rather die."

"If they would rather die," said Scrooge, "they had better do it, and decrease the surplus population. Besides – excuse me – I don't know that."

"But you might know it," observed the gentleman.

"It is not my business," Scrooge returned. "It's enough for a man to understand his own business, and not to interfere with other people's. Mine occupies me constantly. Good afternoon, gentleman."

'Decrease the surplus population' is a shocking utterance. But it is the last few lines that are, perhaps, more telling. They expose Scrooge's fundamental belief in personal responsibility and self-interest in determining health, wellbeing and welfare. Those unable to independently improve their own lot must deal with the consequences.

That this point of view appears in an early-Victorian novella might imply it's an antiquated belief. But it remains dominant today, and its articulation can be found among politicians on both the political left and political right.

In 2018, former Secretary of State for Health and Social Care Matt Hancock said: 'We need to do far more to personally take responsibility for our own health'. His 2018 green paper *Prevention is Better than Cure* took the theme further.[38] It focused on 'empowering people to manage their own physical and mental health needs' – a viewpoint that makes health about individual agency, not social or economic circumstance. Boris Johnson has put it in more 'on the nose' terms – penning a *Telegraph* op-ed in 2004 entitled: 'Face it, it's All Your Own Fat Fault'.[39] While in 2004, then Labour's Secretary of State for Health John Reid told the *Guardian*:

> I just do not think the worst problem on our sink estate by any means is smoking, but it is an obsession of the learned middle class . . . what enjoyment does a 21-year-old single mother of three living in a council estate get? The only enjoyment sometimes they have is to have a cigarette.[40]

Reid's argument poses as the more empathetic but remains a caricature of people wedded to the same politics of civil liberty and opposition to state intervention that underpins the ideas communicated by the political right.

FREE SCHOOL MEALS

More recently, debate around free school meal provisions has provided another case study in the power of the personal responsibility paradigm. Reacting to campaign work by Manchester United footballer Marcus Rashford, Kevin Hollinrake MP wrote: 'where they can it's a parent's job to feed their children'. Ben Bradley MP took his argument further:

> Mad world we live in where saying that parents are responsible for feeding their children is now seen as wildly offensive and controversial. Dare I say that a long-term degradation of personal responsibility is part of the problem here? You don't fix poverty with freebies!![41]

There is now formal research that shows the dominance of personal responsibility in public health policy. In January 2021, a study published in *The Milbank Quarterly* by Dolly Theis and Martin White reviewed interventions on the issue of obesity – an area where personal responsibility discourse is particularly prominent – between 1992 and 2020. Their research found that, firstly, (cross-party) policies overwhelmingly make high demands of individual agency and behaviour change. Crucially, they also find that where policies *seem* to break with this and suggest a more interventionist approach, they are overwhelmingly formulated in a way that 'does not readily lead to implementation'.[42]

This is all to expose a major friction that sits at the heart of health policy in twenty-first century Britain. When it comes to medical treatment, we have a system formulated on collective responsibility whereby we all come together to share the cost of extending a comprehensive, modern healthcare system to everyone.

By contrast, the status quo when it comes to public health before a diagnosis is a viewpoint that early, avoidable, or unfortunate cases of illness are a consequence of bad behaviour – rather than the violence of poverty or racism engraved upon our bodies. We are a country that is happy with state intervention to treat the misfortune of illness, but not to address the conditions in which illness occurs.

CHALLENGING PERSONAL RESPONSIBILITY

Evidently, personal responsibility for our health is a tempting notion. In my own work, I hear it surprisingly frequently from people on the left, as well as people on the political right – including at times from democratic socialists who would never openly subscribe to meritocracy.

Just as with developed leftist rebuttals to meritocracy, the most powerful counter is to focus on some of the highly suspect conclusions that personal responsibility implicitly relies on. Namely, that it demands that we believe that Black people, working class people, people living in the North or people in insecure work all experience health inequalities because of a common moral failure.

Take the town of Blackpool. Residents of this seaside resort are about twice as likely as others in England to be admitted to hospital for intentional self-harm. They are also about twice as likely to be admitted to hospital for an alcohol-related health condition. Teenagers living there have a one in three chance of becoming pregnant before the age of 18, compared to a one in six chance in the rest of England. People are more likely to suffer a violent crime, and twice as likely to be hospitalised by that violence than in the rest of England. The obesity rate is twice the England average.

Compare that to Wokingham, a pretty market town in Berkshire, South England. Here, life expectancy is two and a half years higher than the England average. It's far, far less likely you'll die of a serious illness like cancer or heart disease before age 75. There are fewer serious injuries on its roads. Fewer children live in low-income families, the homeless rate is very low and hospital admissions for violence are far rarer than the country's average. If you live in Wokingham, then it is not impossible that you'll experience bad health – or even worse health than a friend or family member in Blackpool. But it is much, much less likely, on every single count.[43]

Inescapably, the personal responsibility hypothesis concludes that people in Blackpool are subject to some moral failure not often found among the people of Wokingham. It does not and cannot entertain the idea that it might be down to the fact Blackpool is one of the most deprived parts of the country. Or the fact that Blackpool's tourist economy has been hit hard in recent decades. Or that its experience of deindustrialisation has hit jobs and communities. Or that 40 per cent of private sector dwellings in Blackpool have been classed as non-decent.[44] Or that austerity has disproportionately hit its local authority and public health budgets. Or that people in Blackpool must contend with fewer jobs, lower incomes and worse education outcomes than people elsewhere.[45]

Personal responsibility is a paradigm with no room for empathy or mitigating factors.

Personal responsibility as a notion can even have negative clinical consequences. This finding has been seen particularly clearly around lung cancer. Research shows that experience of stigma among lung cancer patients – linked to its strong association with tobacco use – can cause anxiety, depression and the severity of physical symptoms.[46] Significantly, this impacts both lung cancer patients who smoked heavily, but also lung cancer patients who have never smoked. Personal responsibility is a health hazard in its own right.[47]

The opportunity offered by the social justice frontier is an expansion of leftist health principles to address the drivers of health need currently outside the remit of the NHS. The opportunity can be conceptualised by thinking about the elements of health that Nye Bevan did *not* include in his conception of a comprehensive health service.

A simple conception of a 'health pathway' might run as follows:

- The conditions in which we live: This covers the variables that define our life and lifestyle, and covers broad social factors like experience of poverty, income, education, employment, relationships, childhood events, low pay, or homelessness.
- A direct cause: Something puts us at causal risk of ill health (smoking, poor diet, lack of exercise, dangerous hobbies, alcohol or drug addiction, low income, problem debt, hazardous housing).
- A symptom emerges: We notice something wrong. Our heart is racing. Our breath is short. We have a pain, or lump, or bump.
- We seek help: In the UK, there are two main access points. First, a General Practitioner, who provides a gateway into the health system itself. Secondly, Accident and Emergency, when the need is more pressing.
- We get diagnosed: Our illness is identified, either by a physical examination, some medical equipment, or so forth.
- We get treatment: ranging from physiotherapy to pain relief, antibiotics, medicine, or surgery.

When he created the National Health Service, Bevan did not create a health service that covered the entirety of this pathway. The NHS intervenes about halfway through – somewhere between the point we notice a symptom and the point we receive a formal diagnosis.[48] That leaves a whole region of space where our health is not supported by a publicly run, universal system. This is where his principles – universalising the best, free at the point of delivery, based on need, funded by taxation and available to all – are most dearly needed.

THE UNIVERSAL PUBLIC HEALTH SERVICE

The crucial question is this: could the NHS's principles of collectivism and state intervention be extended to social inequality? Can we extend the NHS's brilliance to preventing illness – to taking on the conditions that make people sick – rather than just treating it? The answer is yes, with bold ambition and political will – through a new **Universal Public Health Service**.

In fact, the country has a (tiny) version of this already in place. Local public health services are currently delivered through a ring-fenced grant – 'the public health grant' – and overseen by a Director of Public Health in each local authority. These services are remarkable for being both incredibly effective and extremely cost efficient. To give an example – putting a single pound into local sexual health service budgets comes with a return on investment of £11. For every £1 spent locally on preventing children from starting smoking, we can recoup £15 worth of benefits.[49] One study concluded that public health services are 'three to four times more productive' in producing health benefits than NHS healthcare services.[50]

Despite this, the budget for the public health grant has faced severe cuts during the last decade. My research shows that the budget has been cut by a quarter since 2013/14. Worse, those cuts have almost exclusively come from the poorest parts of the country. The ten least deprived local authorities in England have shouldered just £1 in every £46 cut from local services, while the ten most deprived have put up £1 in every £7.[51]

These are services designed to save the NHS money and, most importantly, avoid people experiencing life changing diagnoses, wherever they can be avoided. Unsurprisingly, the cost of cutting such services was keenly felt during Covid-19 – a disease that thrived in places where underlying health conditions were most common. My analysis has shown that areas that saw the highest mortality rates in the first wave of the pandemic had experienced local public health budget cuts three and a half times greater than areas where Covid mortality was lowest.[52]

Even at their peak, our public health service has never had anything like the firepower needed to fully prevent the vast amount of avoidable ill-health people experience today. Between national and local services, the total budget comes to about £4 billion a year – a pittance on which to run anything like a comprehensive public health system. £4 billion is the equivalent of just 2–2.5 per cent of everything spent on health and social care in England.

A Universal Public Health Service (UPHS) would be about scaling our ambition on state-led public health services by an order of magnitude. It would take forward a very simple principle: if we are willing to collectively pay for cancer treatment when someone gets sick, we should be willing to pay for a social intervention that – based on the evidence – would prevent someone from receiving that diagnosis. Not only would this improve our total stock of health, and make a huge contribution to health justice, it would make our overall health spending far more efficient and take huge strain off the National Health Service in the years and decades to come.

A few models could provide the foundation for this endeavour. Research that aims to identify the root causes of poor health tends to include the following:

- Access to high quality, holistic education
- Access to healthy, sustainable diet
- Good quality employment, pay and occupational health standards
- Financial wellbeing
- Access to good, affordable housing
- Social relationships and community ties
- Access to utilities, such as heating, clean water, and internet
- Fair distribution of income and wealth

In 2021, I published research using the ONS' Health Index that showed – in the most recent data – the most consistent predictors of good health in places included: 1) what happens in our early years and school years; 2) levels of income and wealth inequality; 3) rates and experiences of poverty, particularly in childhood; and 4) the access children have to healthy diets.[53] This indicates where gains can immediately be secured, and where the UPHS should prioritise.

In its first iteration, a Universal Public Health Service could cover each of these. In doing so, it need not be 'one-size-fits-all'. The mission of the Universal Public Health Service should be a) creating an evidence base of social interventions that demonstrably improves health (i.e., equivalent to the medical breakthroughs that provide new drugs); b) allowing local public health experts to seek out need in their local communities (equivalent to diagnosis) and c) ensuring the resources are in place to address those needs, whatever these may be (the equivalent to allocating treatment). In every case, this should be relational – decisions should be made with, not for, people. No-one should be compelled to accept help, in the same way they are not compelled to accept medical treatment.[54] Specific service delivery should be led primarily from places, rather than from Whitehall – recognising that there are very different social priorities, even in places with very similar health profiles. And funding should be heavily weighted towards the most deprived parts of the country, recognising differences like those we've already discussed between Wokingham and Blackpool.

Below I outline what a core offer for such a service could look like when first formed.

Prescription 1: Equal Education for All

Good education is a vital foundation for good, lifelong health. There are some ways where the overlap between health and education is obvious: sex education; a progressive approach to teaching about drugs and alcohol; a school environment that values relationships; the provision of counselling and mental health support. This can all provide a strong basis for a healthy life.

But education that is not 'health education' is just as important (if not more). In 2010, Professor Sir Michael Marmot concluded his report on health inequalities by observing that:

> Inequalities in educational outcomes affect physical and mental health, as well as income, employment and quality of life . . . To achieve equity from the start, investment in early years is crucial. However, maintaining the reduction of inequalities across the gradient also requires a sustained commitment to children and young people through the years of education.[55]

Elsewhere, education disparities have been linked to very tangible health injustices. Children with the best education are estimated to have a life expectancy four years higher than those with the worst, by the time both are aged 30.[56]

The universality of the UK's education system has never been more at threat. One of the clearest examples of this are the rising rates of exclusion from school. Having fallen at the start of the century, the last decade has seen a perilous rise, with 8,000 children excluded permanently from school in 2018/19. In the same period, over half a million children had a fixed-period exclusion – a rise of 25,000 in a year.[57]

Overwhelmingly, these exclusions impact people from minority ethnic backgrounds. People who identify as part of the traveller community have a one in five chance of experiencing an exclusion; Black Caribbean children have a one in ten chance, and white British children a one in twenty chance.[58] Those children are more likely to experience severe psychological distress in the immediate aftermath of the event.[59]

Elsewhere, there is the pernicious practice of 'off-rolling' – whereby a school removes a pupil without recourse to a formal 'permanent exclusion' (i.e. by pressuring the parent to remove their child).[60] In 2019, as many as 49,101 students simply disappeared from school roll. A disproportionate number are from 'Black ethnic backgrounds' according to figures from the Education Policy Institute.[61]

Exclusion is not guaranteed to impact the long-term health of children. But it does immediately and significantly increase the risk of worse long-term health outcomes. Beyond exclusions, there are severe attainment gaps across and within our schools. By the time they finish their GCSEs at age 15 or 16, the most disadvantaged children will be a year and a half of learning behind their peers.[62] The attainment gap is only likely to widen in the aftermath of Covid-19. Research before the pandemic showed that time away from schools – like the summer holidays – widens the education gap between the most and least affluent children.[63]

The impact of 2020/1 school closures, combined with insufficient catch-up funding, is therefore very likely to cause significant inequality.[64]

One of the key levers intended to address educational inequality in England is the 'pupil premium' – through which extra funding is allocated to schools serving eligible children. In principle the policy is a good one – it allocates resources to the poorest in society, at a point early enough in their life to make a major difference. In practice, however, the premium has not narrowed the attainment gap.

The problem is one of coverage and of scale. Currently, a state secondary school will receive £955 a year – less than £3 a day – to address the impact of deprivation on a child's education.[65] A primary school will receive a little more: about £1,345 per student, or just £4 a day. For even these small sums of money, there is no mechanism to reliably ensure the funding benefits the child who needs it. Indeed, secondary schools in the most deprived parts of England saw their budgets cut by about 13 per cent between 2009/10 and 2019/20 – compared to a 9 per cent average cut – making pupil premiums little more than lip service.[66]

It makes for a woeful comparison to the advantages the most affluent parents can provide their children. Average private school fees now stand at £17,000 per year.[67] That might then be topped up further – through school trip fees, sports equipment, extra tuition, after school clubs, or musical instruments. Put in these terms, it's unsurprising that the evidence shows wealthy children outperform talented children in the educational system.[68]

Given how conclusive the evidence is on the link between education and health throughout our lives, any lack of sufficient education investment is a classic case of short-sightedness. It makes little sense if we simply pick up the tab in healthcare costs later. For that reason, the Universal Public Health Service should introduce a bigger and more targeted pupil premium package, based on giving the most disadvantaged children access to private school advantages within the state sector.[69]

Delivery could work as follows. A local public health team could work with schools in their area to identify where educational needs are greatest. They could then work with children and their families and carers to establish what their priorities and ambitions are. Then the public health professional could put in place a package of financial support that revolutionises that child's education. By working alongside families, teachers and school administrators – to create a personalised and funded education plan – the issue of targeting the support at individual children would be immediately corrected.

In terms of resourcing the prescription, tripling the resource available – and ensuring it is far better targeted – would revolutionise the ability of education to provide every child the best foundation for a healthy life. At an outlay of £7.2 billion per year, public health professionals would have around £4,000 available to support the education of our most deprived primary school children. That early investment would be recouped not only through healthier adults, who make less use of the health service, but through a stronger, fairer economy.[70] The interventions funding through the premium need not be aggressively focused on attainment. It might be that money is not best targeted at extra tuition, but at providing counselling, speech and language therapy, nutritious lunches. The latter better align with what parents and children currently think schools most need.[71]

The importance of holistic opportunities suggest we should take this prescription one step further. Children in the most affluent families have access to any number of hobbies – music, sport and art. Again, this is good for health. Not only does participation in extra-curricular activities help academic outcomes, but they also immediately boost a child's health. The most recent evidence shows that ability to participate in an extra-curricular hobby increased levels of optimism and life satisfaction, and reduced depressive symptoms and levels of anxiety.[72]

For £720 million per year, the state could provide the Universal Public Health Service with the means to 'prescribe' every child on free school meals a hobby of their choice – and recoup those costs through better childhood mental health. This would clearly be timely. A childhood mental health crisis is one of the clearest legacies of Covid-

19. One indicative study found a 44 per cent increase in symptoms of depression and a 26 per cent increase in PTSD among eleven–twelve-year-olds during just the first national lockdown.[73] While it is important the NHS is there for them, public health interventions like this one could stop that need from either developing or worsening.

Prescription 2: Nutritious, Free Meals to End Food Poverty

In October 2020, the Queen's birthday honours included an MBE for twenty-two-year-old Marcus Rashford. Earlier in the year, he had won a significant victory on his campaign for free holiday meals for school children. The award of the MBE did not put any halt to his campaigning. Just days later, he restarted his campaign in reaction to a decision by the UK government not to extend school meals to April 2021 in England. Scotland, Wales and Northern Ireland had, by contrast, chosen to maintain provision.

Food insecurity is a major and multifaceted problem in Britain today. Even before Covid-19.3 million children were at risk of holiday hunger, which can cause severe emotional distress, including trauma; can lead to physical health problems because of malnutrition; and can lead to worse educational outcomes, the importance of which we have just covered.[74] But in modern Britain, the consequences of food insecurity also go beyond hunger. A combination of rising prices for healthy food – and an increase in the accessibility of cheap, unhealthy food – means obesity, hunger and malnutrition often go hand in hand. Around two thirds of adults are overweight or obese, childhood obesity has reached record levels, both adult and child obesity is more common among people living in poverty, and has direct causal links to cancer, coronary heart disease and Type II diabetes.[75]

A Universal Public Health Service would allow us to implement a very simple solution: free nutritious food, for everyone that needs it, when they need it. The evidence behind giving people healthy food, when they can't afford it, is compelling. It has been shown to improve security, quality of life and diet.[76] It simultaneously tackles hunger and obesity.[77] It is nothing short of a silver-bullet when it comes to childhood health.

When implemented, free nutritious food schemes have often been highly successful. A scheme called Rose Vouchers run in several local authorities throughout the UK, has shown some remarkable outcomes. The scheme runs as follows: someone in the children's services sector identifies a child or family in need; that child's family is given £3 to £6 per week to spend in open air fruit and veg markets; the family gets better food security and local businesses are boosted. Formal evaluation has shown:

- Children and families using the scheme were happier and healthier
- Families using the vouchers ate less unhealthy food like takeaways
- Families using the vouchers ate more fruit and vegetables[78]

The Universal Public Health Service could simply scale this example of local innovation – by providing a universal healthy food prescription service.

There is a growing movement in support of this idea. In Summer 2020, the IPPR released a cost proposal for a food subsidy of £21, for all children at risk of food poverty. As well as providing better health, food security is also beneficial for planetary health.[79] Calls for a healthy food scheme are part of the final conclusions from the landmark Commission for Environmental Justice.[80] This link between good health and climate will be discussed in more detail in Chapter 5.

Prescription 3: A Right to Healthy Housing

This chapter has already covered the public health consequences of housing in modern Britain in some detail. The relationship between housing and poor health was only accentuated by Covid, as many with insufficient space or poor-quality housing were forced to stay inside for very long periods of time – and to convert their living space, simultaneously, into school and office.

The case of homelessness was particularly acute. In the wake of the Covid-19 outbreak, the government launched the 'Everyone in' operation – providing hotel and emergency accommodation to those who needed it. Though not perfect, the scheme was widely praised by campaigners and charities. It provided proof that homelessness and rough sleeping could be addressed if there is the will to act decisively. However, the political will proved short lived. The second lockdown in the Winter of 2020/1 came without a return of the everyone-in policy – leaving homeless people exposed to a combination of the elements and the pandemic. This was a political choice.

The health consequences of poor housing cannot be disaggregated from the stock and quality of affordable social housing. The number of people living in social homes halved between 1980 and 2010, and has continued to fall since.[81] This has meant many more people entering the private rented sector, which is often unsustainably expensive. According to Trust for London, average rent currently equals 46.4 per cent of the median pre-tax pay in the capital per cent of the average household income – and 24.1 per cent in the rest of the country.[82] Such extensive costs are one of the dominant drivers of poverty, particularly in-work poverty, across the country.[83]

In their outline of a Universal Basic Services offer, a team from University College London explored what a radical upgrade in social housing stock would look like. Their modelling estimated that meeting needs in the UK would require 1.5 million new social houses – provided rent free.[84]

While their case is not anchored in public health per se, the availability of this stock would be revolutionary from a public health perspective. 1.5 million homes would allow the public health service to provide alternative accommodation for those with severe public health hazards in their homes, where a fix cannot otherwise be properly offered. It would provide, immediately, for the 220,000 people experiencing 'core homelessness' in 2019 – i.e., those sleeping on the streets or stuck in temporary accommodation.[85] And it could be used to significantly alleviate over-crowding experienced by hundreds of thousands.[86]

The Universal Public Health Service could provide housing on a social prescription model relatively easily. Local directors of public health would simply need to identify levels of need in their area, and work with national bodies to commission adequate supplies of 'public health housing'. Once built, public health teams would work with local government to allocate housing to those who need it.

Where homelessness has rocketed in the UK since 2010, other countries have managed to make progress against its proliferation. Finland has seen a drop of 35 per cent by using a simple scheme. They give houses to people who need them, through a 'housing first' model. While the scheme initially only targeted long-term homeless people, a subsequent programme has included prevention of homelessness in the remit. Finland is the only country in Europe to have reduced homelessness since the financial crash.[87] By way of comparison, UK homelessness rose by 134 per cent between 2009 and 2015.[88]

Homelessness is not the only health challenge related to housing that this prescription would target, but this is indicative of the idea that the scheme can work. Moreover, it demonstrates how, while evidently not cheap, delivering health improvement through social justice should be a lynchpin of a Universal Public Health Service.

Prescription 4: Ending the Health Costs of Utility Poverty

Utilities are evidently a prime candidate for a 'free at the point of delivery based on need' approach. First, they tend towards monopoly – one national grid, one owner of regional water pipes. This makes it easy to exclude people in the interest of profit. Second, consumers do not have any choice about needing the product. It is not a consumer luxury; it is a human need.

Almost all utilities can accentuate poor health and the conditions that lead to it. I've already talked about heating, but electricity can be another source of significant stress and need across UK households. The price of power has been rising over time. For example, between 2004 and 2010, electricity prices rose by 44 per cent in real terms – vastly outstripping the cost of living.[89] Those on pay as you go meters are the most likely to find themselves cut off from power, pay the most, and are more likely to be struggling financially anyway. It is a factor in embedding poverty, more broadly defined.

Within the bracket of utilities, digital exclusion must also be considered a clear public health priority. As of 2018, 5.3 million adults in the UK still experienced exclusion from the internet.[90] The Centre for Economics and Business Research, an independent economic forecasting and analysis company, has shown that such exclusion comes with tangible impacts. People who are digitally excluded earn between 3 and 10 per cent less than they otherwise would; they are more likely to be unemployed; they likely have a higher cost of living (online shopping is 13 per cent cheaper on average); they miss opportunities to connect with the community; and they spend longer on routine actions (such as online vs. physical banking).[91]

These are impacts that a Universal Public Health Service should concern itself with on a health and quality of life basis. Such unnecessary and avoidable lost earnings, lost employment potential and increased basic costs will impact life chances. Reviews of the evidence have found a conclusive link between money and ill health – both physical and mental.[92]

Digital exclusion also bars people from a range of direct NHS services. The NHS is making an inevitable move towards digital technology. This was accelerated during the pandemic – with a massive reduction in physical GP appointments, a shift to electronic bookings, a large amount of health information moving online and the introduction of large-scale health apps.

Each of these is amenable to policy – namely, giving everyone who needs it free access to the core resources of twenty-first century life.

Prescription 5: Prescribing Against Low Pay and Low Hope

Work has been a consistent focus in this chapter's exploration of non-medical drivers of health injustice. It would be amiss if a founding offer from the Universal Public Health Service did not offer an intervention aimed at employment.

Simply having a job is not a predictor of the conditions needed to live a healthy life in Britain today. I have already covered occupational health, but in-work poverty is a key problem, too. Over one in four households found to be homeless or under threat of homelessness contained one or more people in work, as of 2019.[93] 56 per cent of people (seven in ten children) in poverty in 2018 lived in a working household, compared with 39 per cent 20 years ago.[94] One in seven food bank users are employed or live with someone who is employed.[95]

From a health perspective, this creates a clear case for increased access to training and adult education. More obviously, it makes the case for universal cash payments, provided to those whose income would put them at risk of poverty – and the health harms that have been detailed throughout this chapter.

The skills component could embody an idea that has already begun to generate momentum – a 'skills wallet'. In the 2019 general election, one of the headline pledges from the Liberal Democrats was a 'skills wallet' – providing £4,000 for training and further education at age 25, £3,000 at age 40 and £3,000 at age 55. The costing came to £1.9 billion a year – which the party said could be covered many times over by reversing cuts in Corporation Tax since 2016.[96]

Translating the idea to public health interventions would require some adjustments. It would be available for those who need it, as a prescription against a lack of further education opportunities suppressing their health and creating substantial health injustices. The specifics of the training – where it takes place, at what level and what aspirations it would support could be decided in partnership between the people who receive it and the public health teams who administer it.

The cash payment component of this prescription would essentially constitute a public health minimum income guarantee – designed to bring people up to an independently assessed 'Healthy Income Standard'. This could be based, directly, on existing conceptions of a Minimum income Guarantee.

The basis for the intervention can be drawn from international trials, such as in Finland. There, a pilot scheme saw 2,000 unemployed people given 560 euros per month, with no conditions on how the money would be used. Evaluation shows significant improvements in financial well-being, mental health, cognitive functioning and levels of confidence in the future. Economic security improved. A small increase in employment was observed (compared to those on Finland's existing benefits scheme). Poverty, bureaucracy and administration costs all decreased. The conditions for a healthy, high quality of life were in place and the model was deemed sustainable, indicating it could be taken and translated from an economic intervention to a public health prescription.[97]

The Finnish pilot has often been derided exactly because the impact on employment was not large. The evaluation records that:

> The employment effects of the basic income experiment were measured for the period from November 2017 to October 2018. The employment rate for basic income recipients improved slightly more during this period than for the control group.[98]

This is an unfair ground on which to dismiss the experiment. Until this pilot, UBI had been avoided because it might actively harm employment – by weakening incentives to work. A small improvement in employment amongst the UBI group is, in some ways, a remarkable departure from the previously accepted orthodoxy.

Of course, such public health-led state interventions in the welfare system should not be designed in a way that encourages employers to simply pay their employees less. This is already a dynamic in the make-up of the UK's welfare system. Research from Citizens UK in 2014 found that the taxpayer tops up wages by £11 billion a year – and that low pay amongst just the four big supermarkets (Tesco, Asda, Sainsburys and Morrisons) cost £1 billion a year in tax credits and extra benefit payments. This kind of situation, which essentially subsidises bad corporate behaviours, can be avoided. Ensuring that the public health interventions here do not simply fuel health exploitation at the hands of capital is the explicit focus of the next chapter.

A SILVER BULLET FOR SUSTAINABILITY

In the twentieth century, we experienced a golden age in health. Our life expectancy rose rapidly, as new medical advances beat back long-standing plights on the nation's health. Today, we are doubling down on that same model of care. However, the interventions that are likely to deliver real progress today will probably require a fundamental change in focus from the established model of twentieth-century health interventions. In justifying the idea of social interventions, Alan Logan and colleagues argued in 2019 that:

> [E]ach person/community should be viewed as a biological manifestation of accumulated experiences (and choices) made within the dynamic, political, economic and cultural ecosystems that comprise their total life history. This requires an understanding that powerful forces operate within these ecosystems; marketing and neoliberal forces push an exclusive 'personal responsibility view of health – blaming the individual and deflecting from the large-scale influence that maintain health inequalities and threaten planetary health.[99]

They highlight exactly how personal responsibility in health – like meritocracy in the workplace, individualism in society, consumer-sovereignty in economics – functions. It supports a small-state view, obscuring the influences of vested interests. As we'll explore in the next chapter, it particularly obscures the vested interests of capital.

This made Covid-19 very difficult for the political right. As an infectious disease pandemic, it made it very hard to maintain a personal responsibility paradigm – not least, because the link between who took the 'irresponsible' action and who suffered the consequences was broken. For a small period of time, the government was pushed towards otherwise unimaginable public health interventions such as the furlough scheme and 'Everyone In'– at the kind of scale demanded by the wider, non-pandemic health reality of rising chronic disease. Sadly, they were schemes limited in decisiveness, scope and duration, as ideology adapted and reasserted itself.

The right will now look to do three things. Firstly, they will suggest 'never again' on public health. Second, they will argue that the big state does not and cannot work in the face of health challenges. They will, wrongly, put lockdown at the heart of the coming years of health and NHS strain – when, in fact, it massively reduced the impact of a Covid pandemic fuelled by austerity, neoliberalism and rising inequality. Third, they will look to exceptionalize Covid-19, as entirely different from chronic non-infectious ('non-communicable') diseases – to avoid big public health interventions against major health challenges becoming the norm.

They are wrong on each count. Overwhelmingly, public health interventions protected our health and our long-term NHS capacity in the face of the lack of resilience discussed in Chapter One. Moreover, we can absolutely view non-communicable diseases as a pandemic with very similar dynamics. Only, rather than passing through air droplets, they are transmitted socially, across places and generations, through the unjust structure of our society and the lack of material conditions that still afflict millions. In this light, we need schemes to collectivise risk and meet the health challenge at the same scale as lockdowns and furlough. And fortunately, in this case we do not need more national shutdowns – far more palatably, we need a Universal Public Health Service.

3
The Economic Frontier

In the 1940s, tobacco companies were busy pushing the idea that their products came with a host of wonderful health benefits. One Lucky Strike poster declared '20,679 Physicians say "Luckies are less irritating" . . . your throat's protection against irritation, against cough [sic]'. Camels, a leading brand of the R.J. Reynolds Tobacco Company, went with a similar line: 'More doctors smoke Camels than any other cigarette'.[1]

Major advertising campaigns were a key factor in rising smoking rates in the first half of the twentieth century. Prior to this, evidence suggests that lung cancer had been a comparatively rare diagnosis.[2] Fewer people received a cancer diagnosis at all, and lung cancer made up a smaller proportion of these diagnoses. This changed sharply in the ensuing decades, with one study of men in America showing an increase in prevalence from about 5 in every 100,000 to about 75 in every 100,000 between 1930 and 1990.[3]

The changing epidemiology of such a lethal disease drove an urgent search for the cause, with tobacco a key suspect. Through the 1940s and 50s, the case against tobacco became irrefutable. In the UK, a decisive piece of research was released by Richard Doll and Austin Bradford Hill in 1954. Through a survey of smoking habits among NHS doctors,[4] they presented damning proof of a causal relationship between the number of cigarettes smoked and lung cancer risk.[5]

From here, momentum built. In 1962 the Royal College of Physicians made a landmark recommendation of a major programme of tobacco control; in 1964, the US Surgeon General published a report arguing for the same; and in 1965, the UK government took its first regulatory steps, with a ban on television tobacco adverts.[6]

Despite some public health wins, it's hard to conclude that the industry has been anything other than remarkably successful in defending its product. Big tobacco remains a global powerhouse. The legal tobacco market has sales worth approximately $820 billion per annum, thanks to the 5.7 trillion cigarettes consumed per year by the 19 per cent of the world's population who smoke.[7] In the UK, the tobacco industry attests to tax payments worth over £10 billion per year, employment of thousands and an economic contribution worth over £2 billion/annum.[8]

Moreover, big tobacco continues to post financial results that defy the widely held assumption that it has become an unsustainable industry and will simply cease to exist as consumers and policy makers react to its harms. In May 2021, Imperial Brands – formerly, Imperial Tobacco: the world's fifth biggest tobacco company – reported a £3.6 billion increase in revenue. Finance experts Hargreaves & Lansdown put this above-expectations result down to 'strong pricing and product mix'.[9] Faithful shareholders were rewarded with an increased dividend payment.

Vintage years were toasted elsewhere, too, with British and American Tobacco highlighting 2020 as 'a strong one for BAT's global business'[10] and Phillip Morris International claiming an 'outstanding delivery by the organization'.[11]

Such excellent end of year financial reports translates to disastrous health consequences. In the UK, around 7 million adults smoke and, according to Public Health England, around 78,000 deaths per year are directly attributable to smoking in England alone.[12] That is more deaths than were caused by Covid in England and Wales throughout 2020.[13] Many more people are diagnosed with a serious, long-term smoking related illness such as chronic obstructive pulmonary disease (COPD).[14] Perhaps most alarming is evidence that shows tobacco use is the single largest cause of health inequalities, accounting for as much as half of the difference in 'amendable mortality'[15] between the most and least deprived communities in the country.[16] By 2030, it is predicted that global tobacco deaths will break 8 million per year.[17] This is assuming that Covid-19 does not lead to a smoking boom – which is far from certain. The number of young adults who smoke in England rose by a quarter in 2020, according to research by University College London and the University of Sheffield.[18]

A slow decline in the UK and Western markets has given big tobacco the time it needed to build a sustainable global presence. It is amongst the biggest benefactors, and most aggressive utilisers, of globalisation. Indeed, despite the industry's negative image in much of Europe and North America, systematic reviews show they have actively positioned themselves as good corporate citizens elsewhere.[19] Taking the global view, the industry now looks as big and strong as it ever has.

At times, the tobacco industry has been able to use some unbelievable methods to avoid regulation. In some cases, they've gone as far as manufacturing and sustaining black markets, by oversupplying cheap tobacco to neighbours of regulating countries in an attempt to undercut their efforts.[20] In one case, reacting to a ban on cigarette imports in Vietnam, British and American Tobacco set up a Cambodia outfit to smuggle cigarettes into the nation – using legal trade flows to mask their illegal smuggling operation.[21] This bypassed legitimate tobacco control policies, for profit – and allowed BAT, whose role in the contraband was not known, to point to the presence of a black market in lobbying the Vietnamese government to open up a legitimate market. After six years, Vietnam caved and rowed back on their tobacco control approach, demonstrating the power of capital to profit from health can defy even national sovereignty.[22]

THE 'BAD EGG' FALLACY

The severity of the health impacts of extravagantly unhealthy industries like big tobacco – and the aggressive tactics used by its lobbyists, at home and abroad – often mean it's highlighted as an exceptional, rather than archetypal, case of health exploitation. This exceptionalisation of a small number of industries in public health advocacy is something I call the **bad egg fallacy**.

The bad egg fallacy views the exploitation of our health for profit by the very worst businesses and sectors as exceptions to the rule. They are framed as people and companies doing something that they're not meant to, as opposed to exactly what all the economic orthodoxies demand they do.

The more difficult truth is that the economic status quo not only accepts businesses that harm our health – it incentivises and demands they do so. Profit at the expense, and through the exploitation of, health is a ubiquitous part of current economic and corporate orthodoxies. As such, any critique of individual businesses which is not couched in the terms of political economy or critique of our economic orthodoxy constitutes – mostly unintentionally – to a dangerous obfuscation of this fact. It communicates the idea that a minority are ruining it for the majority, rather than the reality that the orthodoxy is broken, or that the rules of the game are stacked against the health of the many.

There's no single figure on how much national or global profit rests on health exploitation. But a thought experiment suggests it happens at an immense scale. If we were to imagine an index of all the corporations who profit in some way from poor health, it would certainly include the obvious candidates: tobacco, alcohol, sugary drinks, fast food, confectionery and gambling products. It would also include companies at the heart of climate change, whether fossil fuel companies, or those with large carbon footprints. It would include social media companies, for their impact on mental health. It could cover fashion, beauty and cosmetics sectors, for the same reason. It would cover a whole host of companies with poor records on occupational health and workplace equality – gig economy leaders (Deliveroo, Uber), those with famously poor workplace standards (Sports Direct, Amazon), and those who undermine worker rights, through schemes like Fire and Rehire (from British Gas to Weetabix). It would also include companies that inflict long working hours, stress, or unequal pay on their workforce; those in advertising and product design and those who provide help to any of the above with their strategy, promotions, or branding.

In short, it would cover nearly every major corporation going. There are very few businesses whose profits do not come with some net health cost to the population, albeit of varying scale. This suggests we need campaigns and policies that look beyond the individual bad practice of the worst offenders. Instead, we need to look at the dynamics of the exploitative relationship between capital and health.

This is a challenging fact for the nature of our public health campaigns. Our most visible and best funded public health campaigns are almost always quite targeted. Recent examples include minimum unit pricing of alcohol, increased taxes on tobacco, plain packaging of cigarettes, limits on fixed odds betting terminals, a crackdown on 'loot boxes' in online games or a crackdown on adverts for junk food to children on TV and online. It is very hard to find a public health campaign that anchors itself around a macro-critique of the economic orthodoxy, rather than a micro-critique of the practices of a small number of businesses or an individual sector.

There are some instances where ideas and slogans have suggested a broader focus, particularly in distinctly left campaigns. But closer inspection often exposes superficiality. 'People before profit' is one good example that often appears in the health sector.[23] The words suggest a broad critique of our economic model, and its enablement of poor health.

But, when used in the health context – even in the diversity of its use by a range of public health and radical campaign groups – this idea is almost always targeted at individual sectors and business practices: most often the pharmaceutical, health insurance or direct health provider businesses.[24] In its narrow focus, it fails to provide a genuine, conceptual challenge to the economic orthodoxy. We can trace through some specific examples of this in practice.

In the US, Bernie Sanders has been one of the longest standing proponents of 'people before profit'. In his final debate with Joe Biden during the 2020 Democratic Primaries, he argued:

> If you want to guarantee quality health care to all, not make $100 billion in profit for the health care industry, you know what you need? . . . You need to take on the drug companies and the insurance companies.

Here, as elsewhere, Sanders makes clear that people before profit is a critique of two or three sectors – not a full critique of health's position with our economic model.

Similar examples can be found in UK politics and campaigns, as well. In the months before the 2019 general election, the Labour Party released the policy document *Medicines for the Many: Public Health before Private Profit*.[25] The document focused, almost exclusively on one sector: pharmaceutical companies. It outlined a comprehensive plan to bring more public control over R&D, drug prices and medicine manufacture. That is, it was another example of the language of broad economic critique being betrayed by a narrow focus on one sector.

Problematically, the sectors chosen as the focal point of the left's critique are almost always those explicitly within 'healthcare'. This is another example of the NHS forming the single horizon of how big and bold we're currently willing to be when it comes to radical health.

This chapter is not an apologia for individual businesses or sectors that find themselves held to account or shamed because they make a negative contribution to the sum of the nation's health. Rather, it's an argument that very targeted micro-economic critiques of individual businesses and sectors are simply not radical enough to generate the level of progress we need, and which is possible. At best, such critiques constitute incrementalism.

While the pursuit of small gains is a sometimes sound strategy, the last 100 years should have provided proof that major victories for health – at least, victories that would go against the interests of capital – rarely emerge from an incremental approach of targeting the worst corporate offenders 'one at a time'. I've already highlighted our difficulties in putting the tobacco industry to bed. Even more alarming is the emergence of equivalent public health threats – i.e., those that cause epidemic level health consequences, which market their products aggressively and which use 'tobacco tactics' to lobby against public health measures – in other categories.

Big food and drink are behind a doubling in global adult obesity and at least a quintupling of childhood obesity in the UK since the 1980s.[26] Alcohol and opioids are tangibly slowing life expectancy in the USA.[27] Study after study shows gambling addiction figures may be far worse than thought, with ever more severe mental health impacts being recorded in recent research.[28]

We need to break out from our current game of 'public health whack-a-mole' – where, as one threat is suppressed (very slowly, and with huge collective effort), a new one emerges. We can only bypass this with a more fundamental critique, and with broader, more ambitious and more conceptual policy. This is the opportunity offered by the economic frontier.

HEALTH AND CAPITAL: THE BEVERIDGE REPORT

Moving from a 'micro' (individual businesses) to 'macro' (whole economy) critique means understanding the fundamentals of the relationship between our health and capital. The nature of this relationship defines the value placed on good health, the level of intervention the state is willing to consider to protect health and whether health exploitation by capital is normalised, or even actively encouraged.

The terms of this relationship aren't static. Rather, they evolve and change over time. Exploring these shifts can help us understand how the value of health is bound by political and economic norms. As the origin of modern welfare, the 'Beveridge report' provides perhaps the best place to begin.

William Beveridge's best-selling policy report *Social Security and Allied Services* (1942) defined the design of the British welfare state, including through the recommendation of the formation of a health service. It is sometimes noted that William Beveridge was an unlikely founding father for such a significant expansion in welfare. For a short time a Liberal MP,[29] then a Liberal peer, Beveridge was not always a man with whom state intervention sat easy. While the report for which he is almost exclusively now known was highly interventionist, Beveridge went through long periods of fierce opposition to a large and active state. As Margaret Jones and Rodney Lowe note in their book on British welfare, Beveridge was even uncomfortable with the very word 'welfare':

> Even the supposed founder of the welfare state, Sir William Beveridge, disliked the 'Santa Claus' – or the 'something for nothing' – connotations of the term [welfare]. He preferred 'social service state', which emphasised not just social rights but also individual responsibilities.[30]

Any reluctance Beveridge had was eased by what he believed welfare – including health provision – could offer the market-based economy. Beveridge saw a state-backed health offer as integral to building a thriving and productive economy following the massive destruction of the Second World War.

> The first principle is that any proposals for the future, while they should use to the full the experience gathered in the past, should not be restricted by consideration of sectional interests established in the obtaining of that experience. Now, when the war is abolishing landmarks of every kind, is the opportunity for using experience in a clear field. A revolutionary moment in the world's history is a time for revolutions, not for patching.
>
> [. . .]
>
> The third principle is that social security must be achieved by co-operation between the State and the individual. The State should offer security for service and contribution. The state in organising security should not stifle incentive, opportunity, responsibility; in establishing a national minimum, it should leave room and encouragement for voluntary action by each individual to provide more than that minimum for himself and his family.[31]

The final paragraph is telling. The idea of 'security for service and contribution' suggests a welfare system predicated on supporting to the extent workers can do their duty within markets – and indeed, conditional upon it. The idea of a national minimum, with room for *every* family to provide more than that, suggests a preoccupation with incentives and competition integral to the running of markets. Health and welfare for

Beveridge were valuable for what they could provide in terms of market sustenance and productivity.

Put another way, health was a *means to an end* in the Beveridge report – where the end was thriving markets and productive employment.

A treatment-orientated National Health Service[32] has proven to be an ideal intervention if the objective is to support markets with increased human capital. As an acute service, it does not constrain markets, or force them to consider health as part of some sense of social purpose. It does provide them with a boost, in the form of a healthier workforce ('human capital'). As an intervention, it has helped deliver huge health improvements – but improvements that have plateaued at the point the average person can expect to maintain 'reasonable health' until almost exactly the age of retirement, and to live in below reasonable health thereafter.[33] That is, the length of the average healthy life has now plateaued at the age 'service and contribution' – normally – end.

HEALTH AND CAPITAL: THE AUSTERITY DECADE

This political relationship between health and wealth has evolved from the relationship prescribed by William Beveridge in the 1940s. If health is a means to an end in the Beveridge Report, there has been a fundamental reversal today. The norm in 2020s Britain is not that good health is the basis for a good economy – but that output growth is the fundamental basis, and condition, for good health.

At the turn of the 2010 decade, there was rhetoric suggesting that concepts like health, wellbeing and quality of life would be prioritised over overly blunt considerations like growth. On 25 November 2010, David Cameron gave a major speech on wellbeing:

> But I do think it's high time we admitted that, taken on its own, GDP is an incomplete way of measuring a country's progress. Of course, it shows you that the economy is growing, but it doesn't show you how that growth is created . . . Let me give you some domestic examples, if you like, of this issue . . . We've had something of a cheap booze free-for all – again, supposed to be good for growth, but were we really thinking about the impact of that on law and order and on wellbeing? We've had something of an irresponsible media and marketing free-for-all – again, this was meant to be good for growth, but what about the impact on childhood? It's because of this fundamentally flawed

approach that for decades Western societies have seen the line of GDP rising steadily upwards, but at the same time, levels of contentment have remained static or have even fallen.[34]

In some very isolated instances, there was some policy consistent with this fleeting embrace of wellbeing. Putting cigarettes behind screens was implemented in shops and supermarkets, despite being unpopular with right wing think tanks and the big tobacco corporate lobby. Less successful were short-lived plans for a 'Pasty Tax', which became one of George Osborne's more embarrassing U-turns.

Overall, the policy impact was marginal at best. The associated data, the ONS' national measure of well-being is flimsy, rarely cited and has little to no bearing on decisions. In retrospect, the wellbeing rhetoric did little more than provide a convenient distraction from the fact that austerity represented a fundamental reinforcement of growth as our predominant goal, and GDP as our dominant metric.

With hindsight, David Cameron's focus served as little more than a distraction, for the public and media, from an obsessive preoccupation with output growth. His first speech as premier was titled 'Transforming the British economy: Coalition strategy for economic growth' and mentioned the word 17 times further.[35] Growth was made synonymous with recovery. The plank that linked growth with austerity for the Cameron regime was the idea that public spending either inflates debt or increases taxes, suppressing growth. It is a logic that suggests public spending cuts are necessary to support prosperity.

The idea was enacted with relish. Between 2010/11 and 2014/15, the Department of Communities and Local Government (now the Ministry of Housing, Communities and Local Government) saw a real change in its budget of around minus 50 per cent. The Department of Work and Pensions saw a reduction of 30 per cent. Almost as hard hit were the Departments of Justice; Culture, Media and Sport; Environment, Food and Rural Affairs; as well as the Home Office.[36] The NHS was subjected to one of the greatest funding squeezes in its history, leading it to the brink of collapse by the end of the decade.

The point is this. Austerity's starting point was that growth in output measures, like GDP, should be the ultimate goal of policy and the economy. It also proposed that cuts to public spending were crucial both to maximising growth and ensuring that growth was sustainable (a view, needless to say, that has been entirely discredited since).[37] That means that, according to austerity, cutting health and wellbeing budgets were the best way to improve national health and wellbeing.

In 1948, Beveridge saw health investment as critical to sustaining the market-based economy after a major crisis: a means to an end. In the 2010s, austerity positioned health investment as a deflator on prosperity. Our health was framed as a *luxury* product – one that could rarely be afforded and, even when it could, was unlikely to be the optimal place to put our money. Put another way, the 1940s notion that our prosperity is conditional on our good health transformed to one that suggested good health is conditional on growth in economic output.

ALIGNMENT WITH ECONOMIC ORTHODOXY

In many ways, the transformed positionality of health from Beveridge to Cameron reflects a change in the economic orthodoxies since the 1940s and the 2010s. It is consistent with the transition from a broadly Keynesian to a broadly neoliberal economic consensus.

In her book *Doughnut Economics*, Kate Raworth documents how modern economics became obsessed with growth.[38] From the creation of the 'Gross National Value' measure by Simon Kuznets in the 1930s, she traces how traditional economic models have developed to support the idea that growth in GDP is the objective goal. A range of organisations have emerged to support, embed and normalise the idea (the OECD, Bretton Woods) – and the kinds of simplified, imperfect models and graphs that dominate orthodox school and university economic textbooks work to much the same effect. The right's ability to create a political reality where health is conditional on GDP further supports this transition, and reiterates the idea of GDP as a sole goal of society and the economy. In turn, it supports and strengthens the grip of a neoliberal political economy.

Raworth also points out that we haven't always made prosperity and growth synonymous. Twenty-first century economists have a choice about the world they want to create, and that doesn't have to be one organised exclusively around output growth. In her words: 'For over half a century, economists have fixated on GDP as the first measure of economic progress, but GDP is a false God waiting to be ousted.'[39] That is, we have a choice about whether we want to accept health's subordination to GDP.

When considering about this, we should begin from the realisation that output growth measures like GDP are very poor metrics. In a speech to students in Kansas, John F. Kennedy famously critiqued the limitations of such measures:

> Our Gross National Product, now, is over $800 billion dollars a year . . . but the gross national product does not allow for the health of our children, the quality of their education or the joy of their play. It does not include the beauty of our poetry or the strength of our marriages, the intelligence of our public debate or the integrity of our public officials. It measures neither our wit nor our courage, neither our wisdom nor our learning, neither our compassion nor our devotion to our country, it measures everything in short, except that which makes life worthwhile.[40]

Decades later, and the climate movement has created a full body of evidence showing how GDP is not conductive to other societal goals, such as tackling the climate emergency itself.[41] The same is true of health. In Autumn last year, I worked with analysts at Lane Clark & Peacock (LCP) to examine what explained health improvement, and the big health inequalities that exist between regions in England. The biggest correlates were poverty, wealth inequality, income inequality, childhood education and access to sustainable healthy diets. GDP, by contrast, was an almost entirely useless predictor.

There are then two problems with the view that the health should be conditional on output growth (rather than vice versa). First, growth alone does not predict better or more just health outcomes, meaning health won't just improve with GDP improvements. And second, because GDP is such a poor measure of health, policies introduced from the perspective of improving output growth are highly unlikely to be the same policies that would best support health and wellbeing.

In fact, that GDP is a poor measure of good health is only half the problem with the status quo. Equally troubling is the fact that GDP actively values both illness and the activities that generate poor health.[42]

First, it measures the economic activities that make us sick in the first place. Despite the fact that childhood obesity has risen from under 2 per cent in the 1980s (5–10 years olds) to 10 per cent in reception and 21 per cent in year 6 in 2020, junk food production and sales still make a full contribution to GDP.[43] Despite the fact that alcohol-related deaths reached record levels in 2020, the alcohol market still makes a full, unweighted contribution to GDP.[44] Despite the fact problem or addiction gambling has reached more than 2 million in the UK, gambling is still counted uncritically within GDP.[45]

This ill health is then counted a second time. In the most recent accounts, approximately 5 per cent of the UK's GDP was linked to healthcare expenditure.[46] This means the volume of treatments, diagnostics and other operations all contribute to GDP figures. If an unhealthy product puts us in hospital, that's double bubble as far as GDP is concerned. But if regulation keeps someone out of hospital, by making it harder to proliferate unhealthy products, GDP feels the cost two-fold – in the reduced business activity, and in the reduction in avoidable acute healthcare treatments and services.[47]

So the status quo relationship between health and the economy perpetuates three things. First, it (wrongly) implies that growth is the best way to improve health, supporting the orthodox dominance of GDP (and similar measures). Second, and in turn, it thereby props up measures that do not value health and actively value poor health (both the economic practices that cause poor health, and the resulting hospital activity). Thirdly, it incentivises a health model where a) very little is done to encourage corporations to create good health and b) very little is done to support good health before a diagnosis, in line with the principles of Chapter Two.

The cost of this entirely sub-optimal approach to health falls not on the wealthy, nor on the corporations who profit from poor health, Rather, it falls on taxpayers and the state. The former chief executive of the NHS in England – Lord Simon Stevens – put it well in 2015:

> Because we have a tax-funded National Health Service in this country, rather than employer-based health insurance like the French or Germans or Americans, we don't saddle business with the costs of health care.[48]

If companies make us sick, we pick up the bill – collectively as taxpayers. Executives and shareholders only reap the profits. And that means, at least to some extent, our proud system of publicly funded and universal healthcare has been transformed into a subsidy on those who exploit our health for profit.

Moreover, the costs of poor health are extensive. Recent modelling shows that obesity – among just the current cohort of children – will cost almost half a trillion to the NHS and wider society, over the course of their lives. Childhood mental health will cost £120 billion per year by 2040.[49]

If we don't change this reality, everything else in the rest of this book becomes much harder to deliver. Each chapter, except this one, outlines steps towards a state intervention for radically improving our health. Yet, if those simply subsidise poor business behaviours – or worse, create space for or incentivise new sites and types of exploitation – their impact will be limited, and the political appetite for radical change reduced.

A recalibration of the health/wealth relationship isn't just important in its own terms, it is integral for the integrity of the vision put forward in this book more widely.

NOT A BINARY CHOICE

We needn't see this as a choice between Beveridge's and our modern conception of the health/capital relationship. That would be a false dichotomy. Though Beveridge's conception is evidently preferrable, it has its own limitations.

Beveridge's conception of the relationship between health and economy can be critiqued from a few different perspectives. Feminist critiques of the Beveridge report are particularly well known.[50] In looking to maintain the economic status quo, the interventions pre-scribed by Beveridge were often a reflection of the patriarchal norms of the 1940s. In ignoring gender as a unit of analysis, his work and the policy it influenced allowed existing and repressive power relations to be reiterated. Alarmingly, Beveridge's report actively distinguishes between men and women – and makes its proposals explicitly dependent on the idea that women will contribute disproportionately to welfare, by pro-viding unpaid labour, social reproduction and care.

For Beveridge, the role of the state and the married woman was to enable the productive, economically active and employed working-age man. That this was the dominant consideration in the origin and struc-ture of welfare, and by implication the NHS, continues to have a bearing on healthcare today. This is reflected in the rates of misdiagnosis of endometriosis, and well documented reports of women being told their symptoms are trivial. It is reflected in how the 'hysterical woman' arche-type has underpinned a reluctance to provide pain relief for women having coil fittings. It is epitomised by the exclusion of women from historic medical research on the basis that their hormones might impact the science.

There are equally strong critiques of the Beveridge report's focus on productivity by disabled rights campaigners.[51] Beveridge's schemes, which assume the role of welfare is to get people into work, anchor the kinds of discourse which split the country into 'scroungers' and 'shirkers' – a dynamic taken up and politically exploited by the Cameron/Osborne axis. The focus on productivity gives little scope to unconditionally valuing social justice, nor does it consider how discrimination, or a lack of tailored support, might make it harder for disabled people to access work – beyond the one-size-fits-all welfare package prescribed.

The explicit focus on productivity within the welfare state, as well as the inattention played to power dynamics by Beveridge, means services were and remain primarily designed around the needs of working age, able-bodied white men.

Critiques of Beveridge withstanding, we can still quantify the cost of a move from the kind of system he implemented, to a more brutal and small state version during austerity. This cost can be put in both economic and human terms. The redefinition of public spending on public health as unhealthy saw the UK's ability to prevent good health stall. This departure from our previous trajectory has cost over 130,000 lives, by best estimates.[52] Other research shows economic harm. In early 2018, a team led by Professor Clare Bambra found that a third of the productivity gap between the North of England and the rest of England was explained by disparities in health. They concluded that closing this gap would add £13.2 billion to the economy in just the first year.[53] My estimates in 2020 suggest the economic value of closing this disparity has risen further: to £20 billion.[54] That's approximately twice the gross value added to the economy by the whole of UK agriculture.[55]

We need not be bound to models that came before. The potential for transformative change is for improvements beyond merely readopting a Beveridge model. The specific opportunity is to go beyond the view of health as only valuable insofar as it is good for capital and markets, or the view that it is a luxury good that cannot be afforded because it suppresses capital and markets, to instead view health as a key societal objective and measure – an end in and of itself.

PROTECTING HEALTH FOR THE MANY

Understanding the role it plays within current economic orthodoxy opens up huge opportunities for improving our health. In particular, there are three breaks from the past we can and should look to make:

- We need to allocate health a value in its own right, in contrast to both the Beveridge and Cameron conceptions, which subordinate it to suspect economic orthodoxies.
- We need a target that captures the value of good health and poor health, in a way GDP does not.
- We need a system to transfer liability for poor health created by capital, onto capital itself.

Based on these criteria, there is a strong case for a new target that values health in its own right, and takes aim at the current scope for health exploitation. We might call this a **Public Health Net Zero** (PHN-ZERO) target. Broadly conceived, PHN-ZERO targets a state where it is no longer possible to profit from poor health – an enactment of 'people before profit', for the whole economy.

PHN-ZERO provides an immediate decision point – should we endorse highly interventionist government policy and regulation, or give businesses the chance to set voluntary targets and Corporate Social Responsibility (CSR) schemes? It is important to be clear from the outset that CSR rarely sustains the radical changes needed to properly protect our health. PHN-ZERO cannot be left to shareholder whims or voluntary targets.

Sometimes, voluntary schemes simply do nothing. In the last few years, Public Health England have overseen a 'challenge' from government to the food and drink industry – to remove 20 per cent of the sugar from foods that contribute most to children's sugar consumption. The hope was that the market and the sector could solve the problem themselves, without any need for state intervention. However, since the challenge began in 2016, they have managed to remove just 3 per cent of sugar.[56] It has been little more than a distraction.

In other cases, CSR schemes have provided yet another tool for health exploitation. A 2020 paper led by Mark Petticrew found corporate social responsibility materials from the alcohol industry were chock-a-block with 'dark nudges' – behavioural cues which are designed to encourage people to take actions not in their self-interest – which acted to normalise and encourage drinking.[57] For example, the first sentence of an industry CSR leaflet about the link between alcohol and cancer:[58] 'There is no scientific consensus on why some people develop cancer and some don't'.[59] This sows needless uncertainty: there is strong consensus among the scientific community that differential alcohol use is one reason some people develop cancer, and some do not.[60]

The target of a PHN-ZERO would need to be actively delivered through state intervention, and actively managed by government – specifically, by a new, empowered arm or office within government, with extensive public health powers. I suggest a Government Public Health Unit, located in the Treasury – and with a Cabinet Level Minister, who should report on progress and new policy on an annual basis (as per the Chancellor). The rest of this chapter outlines three effective, evidenced and proportionate powers this unit should have in pursuing a PHN-ZERO, and in ensuring our health is valued in its own right and protected from the worse instincts of capital (*Table 3.1*).

Table 3.1   Proposed Powers for a New Government Public Health Unit

Power	Strategy
Fiscal Disincentive	Primary aim, to encourage changes in corporate behaviour; secondary aim, to raise revenue that subsidises direct public health intervention by the state
Regulation	Create liability for actions in areas and markets where tax is unlikely to be an effective mechanism to change business behaviours
Forms of Ownership	For stubborn problems and emerging threats, the ability to introduce new public-health focused ownership models – including state monopoly and common ownership.

Having talked to many, I am of the strong opinion that these proposed powers would be welcomed by most businesses. While a small number stand to lose out, and their lobbyists will make as much noise as they can, most businesses tell me they want a healthier country. They realise they stand to gain from better health. But they don't think they can achieve the scale of change needed on their own. Privately, they want bold government intervention to be enacted, and to create a level playing field.

This is exactly what PHN-ZERO would achieve: a healthier, fairer and more just economic model, that works for the many.

DELIVERING PHN-ZERO

Fiscal Disincentives

The first strand of delivering a policy like PHN-ZERO is shifting the cost of health exploitation from individuals to capital. Fiscal disincentives have proven effective in every instance they've been used to support public health. One excellent case study is the Soft Drinks Industry Levy (SDIL).

Introduced in the 2016 budget, it added a charge of 24 pence/L on drinks containing 8 grams of sugar per 100ml and 18 pence/L on those with between 5 grams and 8 grams of sugar per 100ml.[61] As such, the first benefit of the sugary drinks industry levy was revenue generation. According to official government figures, the levy raised £240 million in 2018 to 2019. Revenue went up in the year 2019 to 2020, to £336 million.[62] That is money that can be invested in health. At the time of writing, the Treasury is still due to announce what it plans to do with what is now £760 million of income – having committed that every penny will be invested in improving the health of children.[63]

Even more impressively, the levy has led to a significant reduction in the amount of sugar in drinks themselves. The brilliance of public health taxes, particularly those that are designed with thresholds as in the case of the SDIL, is that companies are often very reluctant to either absorb the cost (from profits) or pass it to the consumer (in price). In reaction, the vast majority decided it was in their interest to make their product healthier themselves. The average drink captured by the levy has gone on to reduce its sugar content by 43.7 per cent.[64] They did so in the knowledge that choosing to do otherwise would leave them incredibly vulnerable to new, healthier products entering the market – with lower costs.

The third benefit is remarkable, given the prophecies of doom woven by corporate lobbyists between the levy being announced and implemented. It is this: health taxes did not harm businesses. An analysis of stock market returns from soft drinks companies showed that they'd actually experienced long-run growth following the tax.[65] That is, the state pushing them to become healthier improved their business model

– by making them more sustainable, by enforcing innovation, or otherwise raising their profile.

It might come as a surprise that an initiative pioneered under David Cameron's first majority government – and which austerity chancellor George Osborne has named one of his proudest policies – is the first cited in this section. It is of course important to recognise that a sugary drinks industry levy alone is not immune from many of the problems discussed in this chapter – in particular, it is too specific in its aims to change the basis of the relationship between health and capital.

Conservative governments have since shown that this policy is an exception, rather than the rule. In July 2021 a government-commissioned independent report was published entitled *The National Food Strategy*, which recommended scaling up unhealthy food levies to raise £3 billion. With a backdrop of consternation from the ranks of the Conservative Party, the proposal was dismissed out of hand by ministers. Elsewhere, public health policy both before and during Covid has shown how ideologically uncomfortable the right are with the implications of putting public health first – and shifting the onus for health away from the individual onto corporations.

The true test of PHN-ZERO is not whether there are one-off good examples of public health-led fiscal policies – implemented to keep public health campaigners satiated and distracted from more systemic problems. The test is whether it can be targeted towards a more fundamental shift in our economy, to entirely and evenly shift the cost of health exploitation away from individuals and onto capital.

There are a range of places where we can follow sound international examples in fundamentally increasing our ambition. Continuing with the theme of food and drink, for example, the UK could follow Mexico and Hungary's example, and expand the levy on sugary drinks to all unhealthy food and drink. Hungary's version of this tax dates back to 2011, and covers all pre-packaged products with added sugar, chocolates, salted snacks and energy drinks. In just three years, as many as 73 per cent of consumers had reduced consumption of these products – even though most of this tax wasn't reflected in increased prices.[66] Mexico's tax goes further still and covers all foods with greater calorific density than 275kcal/100g. Evaluations again show that diets have improved since the policy was introduced.[67]

PHN-ZERO does not need to be limited to unhealthy goods, like junk food and alcohol. As the previous chapter indicated, there are many business activities that generate poor health outcomes – from renting out homes that aren't fit for purpose, to reneging on occupational health standards, or allowing discrimination and inequality to thrive in the workplace. These are all health-negative activities amenable to fiscal disincentives. Like the Sugary Drinks Industry Levy, their ambition would primarily be disincentivising corporate exploitation and changing business behaviour – with revenue creation a secondary aim.

For example, new fiscal interventions on causes of poor health in the workplace could give much needed teeth to some of the reporting targets recently brought in on equality standards, particularly regarding the gender pay gap. Despite new legislation brought in under the Theresa May government, which required companies over a certain size to report on pay disparities, unfair pay has remained prevalent. In 2020, the median gender pay gap sat at 16 per cent.[68] An investigation the year before had shown that, despite reporting requirements, four in ten big businesses were reporting a widening gender pay gap.[69]

The pay gap is commonly described as a case of economic injustice, but less often as a health injustice. Yet, the discrepancy (and the discrimination that unpins it) does come with tangible impacts on both women's physical and mental health. One study, carried out in America, showed that women paid less for equal work were more likely to experience depression and anxiety, amongst other mental health consequences.[70]

Pay inequality has a snowball effect. According to the Office for National Statistics, British women will earn £263,000 less than their male counterparts over their life.[71] The consequences of this significant discrepancy in wealth accumulation are likely to be particularly pronounced in later life, when a lower salary and smaller pension constitute twin problems. According to the Chartered Institute of Insurance, a woman can expect to have pension wealth worth £35,700 by the time she reaches 65–69. This is a fifth of the average amongst men the same age.[72] This economic vulnerability can lead to a host of socially undesirable and avoidable outcomes – including worse outcomes for longevity and health-state life expectancy.

There is no reason a levy design could not scale the design of existing public health levies. Based on the conception that both health improvement and health justice rely on equal pay, staggered penalties could simply be linked to the final pay gap announced by companies – based on total employee pay. In all likelihood, it would only take a small penalty to drive forward significant change – and given pay gaps tend to be linked to other drivers of occupational injustice, it is almost certain that public health improvements would be observed.

These are just examples of where a large tax-led 'pay or play' approach could begin. In many ways, the specific examples I've given are far less important than the concept – there is huge opportunity for public health taxes to raise money, improve health and create a more sustainable relationship between health and capital.

Regulation

While an expansive regime of financial disincentives is essential to the PHN-ZERO agenda, it is not the complete answer. There are cases where fiscal disincentives will be less effective, or simply more difficult to implement. In these cases, there is an opportunity for the creative use of expanded regulation.

Public health regulation can be both highly effective and incredibly popular. Take for instance the ban on smoking in enclosed public places and workplaces, introduced in 2007. The policy has been effective on its own terms by contributing to lower smoking rates. Just one year after the ban, research in the *British Medical Journal* estimated that there had been 1,200 fewer hospital admissions for heart attacks – with the British Heart Foundation attributing the legislation to this success.[73] But this measure is perhaps most interesting because of its rise in popularity after implementation. Many will remember the fierce debate around the right to smoke indoors, often framed around civil liberty, the economy and the sustainability of pubs. Today, debate has turned into consensus, as 83 per cent now support the ban – including 52 per cent of smokers.[74]

One area where fiscal disincentive may work less well, and this kind of regulation could contribute, is in the digital economy. Digital taxes have proven difficult to administer. First, because tax is paid from the base of manufacture rather than at the point of delivery, allowing digital giants to plant their HQ somewhere with low tax rates ('profit shifting').[75] Digital business models don't comply with national boundaries in the way normal 'brick and mortar' businesses do. Second, digital regulation often relies on international consensus – which proves difficult to arrive at, given certain nation-state's vested interests in maintaining the current status quo (particularly America's). Third, a lack of transparency over profits makes it hard to target and enforce specific taxes on unhealthy practices – a key design element for public health levies. Fourth, the make-up of the digital economy makes it hard to design taxes that genuinely change corporate behaviour, limiting its advantages. And finally, many of the harms that are caused by social media come from activities that are too toxic to be used for income generation (illegal activities such as grooming or harassment, for example).

For PHN-ZERO to be viable, it needs to have the ability to react to these kinds of challenges.

The digital economy is a sophisticated system of health exploitation. On the one hand, there is an element of dependency. Equal outcomes among children depend on digital access – with Covid-19 and school closures exposing the injustice faced by the one million children and families without adequate access to a device or connectivity in their home.[76] But the digital divide is not the only important measure. The ability to safely access a wide variety of platforms – including social media – is vital in terms of ensuring children have access to the networks, digital literacy and other skills they will inevitably need in the future.[77] Indeed, I have already put forward digital as a key component in a Universal Public Health Service (Chapter Two).

This means bans and content filters are unlikely to be adequate solutions. If all children find their digital and social media use restricted, it will leave them playing catch-up in their adult life.[78] And if our solution to inequality is to restrict digital access to the most disadvantaged children, we will exclude them from the skills, social interactions and networks that will define their future outcomes.

Nonetheless, we cannot ignore the public health risks. Cyberbullying and online harassment affect almost one in ten children aged 10 to 15 in England and can introduce severely negative psychosocial outcomes for victims – including depression and anxiety.[79] Social media has also been linked to social isolation, peer pressure and exposure to inaccurate, unsuitable, or dangerous content.[80] Ofcom, the communications regulator, has shown that eight in ten children between the ages of 12 and 15 have at least one harmful online experience a year – in most cases, relating to interactions with other people or interactions with inappropriate content. For 4 per cent, this was material showing child sexual abuse. For 6 per cent, material encouraging terrorism. For 10 per cent, it was cyberstalking; for another 10 per cent pressure to send photos to another person; and for 15 per cent, it was violent or disturbing content.[81]

Often, the very activities that undermine the health and security of children (and adults) prove highly profitable for social media companies.

In some cases, the link between profit motive and harm can be focused on something ubiquitous. For example, a major method of monetising social media platforms is advertising revenue. Those advertisements are often used, intentionally, to expose children to harmful products, or content that would be more explicitly regulated on television. In 2017, I developed two major surveys – the Youth Obesity Policy Survey and the Youth Alcohol Policy Survey – as part of one of the biggest studies of children and young people ever carried out in the UK. A body of analysis emerging from these surveys shows, beyond doubt, that big food and drink and big alcohol companies are using social media platforms to target kids.[82]

There is also profit to be found in less prevalent, but higher harm content. Social media companies exist in ad supported ecosystems. These systems have not been designed to distinguish between harmful and harmless, legal and illegal content. So, when a gunman killed 49 people at two New Zealand mosques in 2019, and live streamed the incident, Facebook drew an audience and made a profit. When children are exposed to sexual material, or return to conversations with someone grooming them, they generate a profit for the platform.

Regulation can enact the spirit of fiscal disincentives. Public health taxes work on a 'play or pay' basis. They do not force corporations to focus on our health. But they enact sufficient incentive that a) it becomes far less profitable not to do so and b) people impacted have the means, through the state, to exact a price for poor health. In this case, legal accountability can enact this principle. For example, a new regulator with sweeping powers could transform social media, by making certain harms criminal, and introducing civil liability for others. Crucially, this should not be limited to a narrow definition, but should extend the full range of opportunities for the health exploitation from which social media companies currently profit.

Regulation could then be based on a transparent duty of care. A basis for this could be the approach taken in Canada to alcohol, where establishments serving drinks have a 'duty of care' to their patrons. This is a law that ensures commercial liability when harm emerges after drinking in a licenced establishment. In 2017, a British Colombia court found a pub 25 per cent liable when a drunk-driving accident left a pedestrian with a brain injury.[83]

The duty of care in Canada works as follows: you owe a duty to patrons not to overserve. If this happens, they are owed a duty – to be kept safe.

The same duty extended to social media would mean people within the commercial environment – i.e., on a social media site – would be owed safety. Standards of safety could be adopted from a range of other countries. In Germany, the NetzDG law (2018) demands all companies with more than two million registered users set up firm procedures to review content complaints with 24 hours.[84] In the European Union, there is a one hour time limit to take down extremist content.

Where that Duty of Care is not maintained, then liability should come into play. This could include the German approach of massive fines or, better still, the approach taken in Australia – where the *Sharing of Abhorrent Violent Material Act* (2019) introduced criminal penalties for social media executives and fines worth up to 10% of global turnover.

Vitally, any scheme must include full compensation for the person impacted (as opposed to the government alone). This would help encourage people to report harmful materials, and ensure the linkage of those that experience health consequences and those who benefit from health reparations.

Ownership Models

Finally, there is a strong case for using ownership models in the pursuit of a Public Health Net Zero. Ownership models and public control are less frequently discussed in the context of public health. However, they are well evidenced, impactful and revenue creating.

There is a particularly strong case for moving away from private ownership models in the case of fiscal/regulatory interventions which aren't working ('stubborn challenges') – or in the case of new products of public health concern ('new threats'). The specific ownership models used could themselves be varied. We could employ public ownership in some cases – with the Public Health Net Zero Unit empowered to bring distribution into direct public control. Equally, it could see the state enact the conditions for common ownership, to ensure certain resources are only used for purposes with a clear societal benefit.

Direct state control of distribution has been incredibly successful in reducing harm in countries that have used it – most commonly, for the distribution of alcohol.[85] In Sweden, the Swedish Alcohol Retailing Monopoly has the sole right to retail alcoholic beverages. Its website declares 'the purpose is to minimize alcohol related problems by selling alcohol in a responsible way, without profit motive'.[86] There are 400 stores and 500 sales agendas, and the country is free from aggressive alcohol advertising.[87] Similar systems can be found in all Nordic countries except Denmark, and in all Canadian provinces except Alberta.

Direct public ownership of a long-standing and hard to control public health threat has proved remarkably successful. A 2017 study found that if Sweden were to privatise its alcohol retail monopoly, alcohol consumption would increase by as much as 31 per cent. All else remaining the same, that increase in alcohol consumption would be expected to increase alcohol-related deaths by 42 per cent and assaults by 34 per cent.[88] As with other public health measures, while people are sometimes suspicous of their impact before they are implemented, large levels of public support and trust generally then follow. In Sweden, the system has 78 per cent support.[89]

In countries that choose state monopoly, the revenue opportunities are significant – and normally greater than from 'duties' on a private system (as in the UK). Because of the elimination of profit margins, and the vast array of tactics beyond price open to a state alcohol operator to control consumption, there are even examples of state monopolies keeping unit prices lower than private competitors *and* generating more revenue for the state.[90]

In the case of alcohol, state involvement tends to have occurred because it has proven a stubborn threat. Alcohol harms have long been clear in society and have proven less than amenable to other public health interventions. This has justified direct action to both maintain the availability of the product, and to achieve a state where its use is balanced – a sustainable relationship between civil liberty and public health. However, the experience of public ownership and state monopoly can provide a lesson in supporting the controlled introduction of new products that may otherwise have public health harms – a method of safely introducing things the market might not be trusted with.

For example, there is now a strong precedent across the world for the legalisation of cannabis. It was legalised in Canada for recreational purposes in 2018; in Georgia following a court ruling in 2018; in 17 US States, and in a host of other countries, provinces and territories. And there is a public health case for legalisation of cannabis, it its own right.[91] At present, criminalisation of drugs has little basis in evidence – and is rightly suspected to be little more than an instrument of targeted coercion and control by the state. A publicly controlled, managed and legal supply chain could reduce arrests, which are disproportionately of

Black people (and themselves a predictor of poor health outcomes, not least because of alarmingly poor standards of prison health).

State monopoly provides a proactive way to restrict the harms of cannabis – through mechanics like price control, limits on shop density and controlled opening hours. In 2019, one study examining the lessons of public health monopolies for the legalisation of cannabis concluded that 'for public health and welfare, public monopolization is generally a preferable option'.[92] Similar support for state monopoly can be found in the wider academic literature.[93]

Moreover, the experience of giving the market control of legalised cannabis in parts of America have shown that it simply funnels profits to the usual suspects – wealthy investors, private equity companies and big business. As Kojo Koram has put it: 'those who have suffered most under the War on Drugs are . . . excluded from the wealth that is being generated in its transition to a legal market'.[94] Just 1 per cent of cannabis dispensaries in the USA are owned by Black people. State control can help alleviate this question of equity.[95]

State monopoly is not the only form of ownership that might help address stubborn challenges and emerging threats. For example, in the case of reaching PHN-ZERO in the digital economy, common ownership might be an option alongside the regulatory proposals I discussed above.

The health harms of the digital economy cannot be entirely separated from its ownership model. A lack of clear ownership rights of personal data means we can be manipulated by digital giants – whether directly, or in passing on sophisticated insights that help personalise products and advertising. That is, without ownership of our data, we have little insight into how it's being used and little control over to what end. We can be influenced to buy unhealthy products through personalised advertisements, which are more convincing and subtler than anything we've ever faced. Our dopamine receptors can be gamed, to increase our screen time and create addiction dynamics in our social media use – good for owners and advertisers, but disastrous for our mental health. Essentially, without ownership of our data, we neither have knowledge of how our data is used, nor power over its purpose and impact.

There is, therefore, a public health case for taking back ownership of data – both to maintain standards and set conditions on the purposes to which it is put by profit-making entities. In this case, the most viable ownership model is not state ownership, but common ownership, through a digital commons. A digital commons positions the state as a steward, not an owner, of the digital economy. Recommendations made by former John McDonnell advisor James Meadway, the Royal Society and the British Academy have all identified the need for such strong stewardship by the state in managing data.[96]

The digital commons is most often proposed in opposition to the two other options for managing the data economy: more competition (e.g. by breaking up monopolies) and more state intervention (e.g. through regulators). The advantage of the commons is that it prioritises the new forms of communal ownership that have emerged in the digital age and helps avoid unnecessary de-aggregation of data – which is exponentially more valuable when compiled.

There is no better body for delivering this kind of curation and stewardship than one focused on public health. As a distinct natural resource, data has been described as the 'new oil' – on the basis that it does not have innate value but can be imbued with significant value in the process of extraction.[97] But perhaps a more accurate comparison of data is 'the new water' – a natural resource we cannot live without, and which has the potential to cause disease and other health consequences if imbued with impurities. A public health approach to the data commons would place a primary focus on preventing harm, ensuring that the full cost and benefit of data's potential is taken into account whenever and whereever it is used.

The power of innovative ownership models for products that we want to safely distribute has been relatively untapped in the UK. Their power to radically improve health should be an integral part of the power of any new public health body, both for raising revenue and for achieving public health gains.

A NOTE ON POWER

PHN-ZERO offers the opportunity to revolutionise health by moving towards a model of active public health stewardship – by the state, in the collective interest and as an expression of a collective will.

This does not come without a need for caution. Public health interventions have long been plagued by accusations of paternalism, today often expressed through the concept of the 'nanny state'. This framing defines punitive interventions as attempts to control people, particularly poor people, based on the moral ideals of the public health establishment.

It would be foolish to suggest there has never been an element of power and control to the work of the public health movement. In the eighteenth century, the temperance movement reacted to the 'gin craze' in Great Britain with moralising absolutism. The founder of the Methodist Church, John Wesley, made the issue entirely black and white when calling both the sale and purchase of alcohol evil. The national debate at that point in time was driven by a desire for order by the middle and upper classes, rather than by any genuine interest in population health.

Equally, there must be a concept that allows us to collectively act in the interest of population health. When it comes to economic justice, the left is rarely timid in the face of exploitation. We do not simply tolerate the harms caused by business models like Bright House and Wonga because of civil liberty and the right of all to purchase consumer goods. We act, because the relationship these companies establish between people and capital is exploitative.

That means we must not be blind where injustice might be a consequence. For example, I have focused on the case study of food and drink, as one where taxation works. But in many cases, unhealthy food is often cheaper than healthy food – and if food prices were to rise it could create real difficulties for people already living in poverty. The onus is for any move towards fiscal disincentives not to constitute a penalty or restriction aimed at people without enough money. It must always be combined with mobilisation of revenue in targeted interventions, like subsidies or the kind of services outlined in the Universal Public Health Service. Indeed, the PHN-ZERO and the Universal Public Health Service could have a wonderfully reciprocal relationship, linking revenue creation with need alleviation.

This is the foundation on which an interventionist approach such as PHN-ZERO is justified. It is acceptable insofar as it eschews moralising and focuses on demonstrable exploitative relationships between health and capital. It is not about bans or absolutism, nor etiquette, morals, or standards. It is about prescribing health a value and prescribing a cost when actors – whether intentionally, or because of the environment in which they are competing – profit from poor health. It is about having the instruments to defend the many.

4
The Social Care Frontier

To date, the damage caused by Covid-19 has been disproportionately concentrated on those who rely on social care support. Throughout the pandemic, care homes were one of the key sites of excess mortality, despite government proclamations of protective rings and emergency funds. The first wave of the pandemic saw 30,000 more deaths among care home residents in England than we would have expected, almost all inevitable.[1] People who relied on care in their homes were also at extra risk – with 3,000 'excess deaths' during the first wave – and found themselves subject to by far the most severe impacts from lockdowns and other restrictions.

Older people, adults living with disabilities and people with long-term health conditions alike were critically let down by pandemic policies and left to cope with significantly greater risk.

However, whilst things were inevitably exasperated by poor government decisions during 2020/1, we must be careful not to erase longer-standing structural problems with how care is organised. The reason our social care system struggles – before the pandemic, and during it – is down to its neoliberal foundations. It is the political economy of care which undercuts its sustainability.

NEOLIBERALISM AND CARE

The post-war Clement Attlee government was very clear about the founding principles behind their National Health Service. It was far less clear about what core principles would sit behind the social care system. At best, the 1948 National Assistance Act gave some sense of what was to be expected from local authorities:

> [they will] provide residential accommodation for persons who by reason of age, infirmity or any other circumstances are in need of care and attention which is not otherwise available to them.[2]

It was here that social care was set on a very different path to the National Health Service.

The clause 'not otherwise available to them' is critical. The implication is that local authorities need only use their budgets to meet the care needs of the worst off, or the very most in-need – a conception that allows a) private sector dominance; b) means testing and fees and c) a system built around intervening on acute need as late as possible, rather than addressing emerging needs as early as possible. Each underpins a problem faced in social care today.

Local authorities did continue to directly provide most care in the years following the act.[3] Indeed, Harold Wilson's government expanded their role to make provision of domestic help mandatory, and to cover home adaptations for both older and disabled people. By contrast, the independent sector remained a small stump, delivering a very small fraction of care services. Nonetheless, the 1948 legislation still allowed for the registration and inspection of profitable care providers; allowed fee charging independent services to be commissioned; and accepted the concept of personal payment for care.

This was a crucial enabler for the radical social care reforms implemented by the Thatcher governments. In general, her governments were very conscious of the problems posed by an ageing population. The projected speed of population ageing promised to place a bigger strain on public services, increasing demand on the state and, in turn, increasing state expenditure.

Nowhere would state expenditure go up faster than long-term care services. So, when they looked to isolate areas where state expenditure could be reduced – including by moving more service provision into the private sector – long-term care was a clear candidate.

The strategy focused on mobilising older people's money (through means tests) into an independent market (created through pump priming with public funds).[4] The approach wasn't a guarded secret. Indeed, in a review of the community care system, Roy Griffiths wrote:[5]

Many of the elderly have higher incomes and levels of savings than in the past . . . this growth of individually held resources could provide a contribution to meeting community care needs.[6]

In the same document, he outlined his central idea of local authorities as 'brokers' of care, not direct providers. He suggested they act as 'the designers, organisers and purchasers of non-health services, and not primarily as direct providers' – that is, he imagined the local authority becoming the equivalent of a travel agent for the package care deals offered up by big private providers.[7]

When it came to creating a market, state resources were the basis for growing and sustaining a dominant independent sector. For instance, between 1980 and 1990, there was an explosion in the use of Supplementary Payment benefit – a form of social security – to fund places in private care homes. The process worked as follows. Previously, local authorities assessed care needs, and then put in plans to meet them. But in the 1980s, a new scheme was formalised whereby people could bypass their local authority's assessment and use national welfare budgets to take an immediate place in an 'independent' sector care home. As Stewart Player and Allyson Pollock have shown, there were just 11,000 recipients of Income Support in private and third sector nursing and residential homes in 1979, at a cost of £10 million per year.[8] By February 1993, the figures had reached almost 300,000 people and a cost of £2.6 billion per year.[9]

This rise is hardly surprising. The 1980s saw a significant squeeze on local government budgets. Many local authority leaders were relieved to have the opportunity to use a central department's budget to fulfil statutory social care duties. In some cases, people were actively encouraged to use the social security system to pay for care in a private sector care home. In others, local authorities engineered bureaucratic assessments, to encourage people to seek much quicker independent sector alternatives.

The *National Health Service and Community Care Act* 1990 followed,[10] enacting Griffiths' idea of a fundamental redefinition of the role of the public sector. Funding for social care devolved from central government to local government. The transition came with a new role for local authorities – as Griffiths has postulated, they became brokers, rather than providers, of care.[11] To ensure dominance of the independent provider sector, and that local authorities did not take the opportunity to deliver better, cheaper care directly, a new Special Transition Grant was made available for personal care, with a stipulation that at least 85 per cent of the money would be spent on private sector providers.[12]

At the time, these reforms were framed as a move towards a 'mixed economy' of social care provision. In reality, it delivered near total dominance of social care provision by the independent sector. In 1979, about two thirds of residential and nursing home beds were provided by either local authorities or the NHS. In 1993, 95 per cent of domiciliary care was provided by local authorities. By 2012, the numbers were 6 and 11 per cent respectively.[13]

NEOLIBERAL CARE TODAY

The care system's neoliberalism has only increased in the subsequent decades. The market share of the private sector continues to tick up year on year. Analysis by the IPPR and Future Care Capital found a 2 per cent increase in private sector provision between 2015 and 2019 (though this might not sound like a huge increase, the increase comes from an existing position of private sector dominance).[14]

As significant as the market share of the private sector is the increasing shift in the market – from small providers, better embedded in the communities they serve, to large providers. As in many other parts of the country's economy, small, family-run providers are being pushed out by large, faceless corporations. The most recent analysis shows that five big providers control almost one fifth of the social care sector.[15] Behind them, the relative market share of companies with fleets of at least 50 care homes is growing, while small companies overseeing one or a few local residential homes are struggling.[16]

The shift to large providers has come alongside a significant shift to provision by firms funded through private equity. At the time of writing, the five biggest companies are: HC-One Limited (5.1 per cent market share); Four Seasons (3.7 per cent market share); Barchester Healthcare (3.3 per cent market share); Care UK (2.4 per cent market share) and BUPA Group (2.2 per cent market share). That gives the five biggest providers control of almost 20 per cent of all for-profit social care beds. Three of these are owned by private equity (HC-One, Four Seasons and Care UK).[17] One more is a public company with ultimate shareholder registration in Jersey, a tax haven (Barchester Healthcare).

This shift from a public to a private delivery model in social care will be, for many, sufficient enough evidence to justify a major and radical reform project. But in making the popular case, it's important to go one step further – and to fully outline how the shift has translated into negative outcomes: for people, for the sector and for workers.

LOW QUALITY, LOW ACCESS, HIGH COST

The shift towards big, private equity funded care provision has come with direct implications for quality of care.[18] There is evidence that private providers offer lower levels of training and lower rates of workforce pay than their voluntary and public counterparts. In turn, they have higher rates of staff turnover and lower overall levels of staffing.[19] Other studies, including one by the sector's inspector, the Care Quality Commission, have shown that a smaller, less well-trained workforce translates to a measurable impact on the quality-of-care provision provided.[20]

It's unsurprising, then, that there is a link between the size of a provider and the quality of care it provides. 89 per cent of small nursing and residential homes have either a good or outstanding rating from the Care Quality Commission. In large residential care homes, the figure is 72 per cent good or outstanding, and in large nursing homes the figure is just 65 per cent.[21] Worse, there are hundreds of care providers that have never had a rating better than 'requires improvement'.[22] That is a remarkable differential in quality of care. It indicates the human consequences of how the social care system has evolved over the last four decades, and also demonstrates how many people could find themselves receiving inadequate levels of support if further shifts to larger, more heavily financialised big corporate providers are allowed to continue.

Poor care is the tip of the iceberg. A lack of public investment over decades in social care has meant, in essence, a system designed only to provide care for those with the very greatest need. Funds only become available when people have deteriorated – when their needs have become far more intensive – rather than when an intervention could still maintain their health and independence.[23] As many as nine in ten local authorities in England only provide care for people who have either 'substantial' or 'critical' needs.[24]

This means there are huge levels of unmet need across the country. In 2018, I released research while at Macmillan Cancer Support that quantified this for the cohort of people living with cancer. That analysis showed that as many as two in three people living with cancer had practical care needs – but that only a fraction was getting adequate levels of support. When asked about the support they needed within their homes, 38 per cent of people on a low income and 19 per cent of people on a high income had unmet needs. When asked about the support they needed outside of their homes, 34 per cent of people on a low income and 13 per cent of people on a high income had unmet needs.[25]

More broadly, a comprehensive review of unmet needs in adult social care by the Centre for Analysis of Social Exclusion found 1.5 million adults living in England and over 65 with at least one unmet care need – leaving them without the support needed to live a good life.[26] Age UK predicts this will rise to 2.1 million by 2030, without intervention.[27] And while there is no equivalent figure for people under 65, analysis by the Health Foundation shows that 35 per cent of the requests made by people aged 18 to 64 are rejected by their local authority.[28]

This underwhelming system comes with a significant cost. Under the current system, people pay until they no longer have assets worth £23,250. This means a great many people lose almost all of their wealth, over the course of their lifetime. According to the charity Independent Age, around 143,000 older people face the prospect of paying 'catastrophic lifetime costs' of £100,000 or more – around one in three people within the residential care system.[29]

It's a hugely regressive system. In essence, it is designed to take *all* the wealth of most, working people who have the poor fortune to need help when they get older – while leaving the finances of the very richest broadly intact.[30] In practice, it operates as a 100 per cent inheritance tax for those with the least money, with the proceeds going into private profits rather than the state. It is a system that keeps the poor, poor and the richest, rich – across generations.

The regressive nature of our social care system looks set to continue. In September 2021, the government announced a 'new plan' for social care. Under this plan, people will pay up to £86,000 for their social care (over their life)[31] – and they'll only pay if their total wealth is under £125,000. This is scheduled to come into effect from Autumn 2023. But this will still leave us with a system that benefits the wealthiest. Modelling of this system has shown:

- A person with a house valued at £125,000, receiving 5 years of social care, would spend 49 per cent of their wealth on care – leaving them at clear risk of financial ruin
- A person with a house valued at £500,000, receiving 5 years of social care, would spend only 17 per cent of their total wealth on social care – leaving their finances broadly intact

That is, even once this new policy comes into effect, it will still mean a social care system that operates on the brutal logic of American healthcare.

CHRONIC PROVIDER FRAGILITY

Another consequence relates to the stability of the providers who deliver services. Indeed, the current private equity-dominated social care system bears comparison to the Private Finance Initiatives (PFI) that were widely criticised when extensively used by the NHS between 1992 and 2018.[32]

The mechanics of PFI worked as follows. NHS trusts would put out a tender, asking for expressions of interest from private sector contractors, to build new health capital assets. These tenders would be for large projects – such as the construction of new hospitals. Bids would then come from consortiums, with successful parties forming a 'special purchase vehicle'. The consortium would then, usually, fund the construction of the hospital using large amounts of debt. The NHS would not face any costs until the build was complete. But once it was, they would begin paying 'unitary payments' – an annual charge that was meant to cover the risk taken by the private sector, but which in reality saw individual NHS trusts pay significantly inflated fees.[33]

The risks associated with this model of public–private partnership were epitomised in 2018 when Carillion – one of the biggest PFI beneficiaries – collapsed. It immediately left behind £7bn of debt, 3,000 lost jobs within the company and a further 75,000 impacted jobs within its supply chain.[34]

While the government have since committed to ending PFI procurement, the problem is not the scheme per se, but the relationship between the state and the private sector it represents – broadly the same relationship that defines the relationship seen in the social care market. As with PFI, here the state underwrites guaranteed payments, supporting large private sector profits. To maximise those profits, social care providers often look to expand through extensive use of debt and other high-risk business practices. The resulting system is defined by its expense to the taxpayer, a lack of quality as the sector looks to maximise profit and a lack of provider stability that often leads to high profile collapses.

Social care has been host to a number of big, 'Carillion-style' collapses. Most recently, the Four Seasons Healthcare provider went into administration, putting the care of 17,000 residents at risk, as well as the jobs of 22,000 employees. In 2011, major operator Southern Cross also collapsed after just 15 years of operation, 9 of which had seen it owned by venture capital firms.

The story of Southern Cross is illuminating. Before its collapse it had been in the middle of a significant expansion. It quickly became the largest operator in the sector. Rapid expansion led to large profits for investors and very generous salaries for the executive team. One executive sold his individual stake in the company for a substantial £36.6 million (550p a share). Just months after this transaction, Southern Cross announced its first profit warning.[35] By July 2011, it announced its closure – news that left the residents of its 752 care homes with a very real threat of homelessness hanging over them.[36.]

The closure comes down to the strategy Southern Cross used to expand as quickly as it did. It had worked on the basis of building properties, selling them off and then leasing them – a concept known as 'sell and leaseback'. As a practice, this is a high-risk, high-reward method of increasing liquidity – enabling expansion. In the end, Southern Cross could not sustain the liquid funds needed to meet its huge running costs – nor could it provide the quality of services needed to retain sufficient resident numbers. That doesn't mean their approach didn't make some people very rich in the meantime. It wasn't investors or executives who lost out. It was workers, service users and the taxpayer.

Southern Cross were not trying to go bankrupt, nor were the other care providers who have failed. Rather, their strategy was to make as much money as possible, as quickly as possible. Those running and profiting from Southern Cross didn't face any of the risk and consequences of such a high-risk strategy. It was the state and care home residents that paid the price of their strategy, designed around profit extraction rather than high quality public service.

Carillion's collapse was equally a collapse linked to a crisis of liquidity, brought about by an unsustainable reach for fast profits. The PFI construction company recycled its own liquidity, by selling its interests in hospitals to investment companies quickly after completing construction – creating funds that could be pumped into expansion and help to maximise profit extraction.

When this instability isn't causing the country's largest adult social care providers to collapse, it can be linked to alarming stories of negligence. An indicative example emerged in at the Whitchurch Care Home in January 2019. A visit from the sector's inspector exposed:

> Widespread and systemic failings . . . during the inspection. The quality and safety monitoring systems used by the provider were not fully effective. They did not ensure that there were the right resources in place to ensure the quality-of-service provision and mitigate risks to people.[37]

Systematic failings include the failure to fix an elevator, meaning second floor residents couldn't be transferred to ambulances; people regularly going without their prescribed medication; and 'occasions when people's dignity had been compromised'.[38] This was a care home being run at the very lowest possible price, under huge financial pressure, trying to remain afloat. In this case, as in so many others, the care providers failed to do so. Whitchurch care home's owner – Four Seasons Healthcare – entered administration three months later.

WORKFORCE EXPLOITATION

While researching this book, I was fortunate to have the chance to hear from social care workers directly about their experiences of working in the sector. During the second Covid lockdown, I talked to Jenny.[39] Jenny had left social care and was happy for her story to be shared.

Jenny had been drawn into social care when looking for a job where she could genuinely help people. Having enjoyed another, short period of employment in the sector – working for a charity in the South West of England – she took a role with a private operator after making a move to London. After just over a year struggling through her role, longer than many others manage, Jenny left the sector altogether.

The first thing Jenny talked me through was the low pay, a universal issue for the social care workforce:

> I was paid about £8 an hour. That's not enough to live on, certainly if you're paying London rent. It cost about £1.50 for the bus each way, and I could end up taking 2 or 3 bus trips an hour.

The base rate of pay is low, but Jenny told me she had at least known this was the case when she accepted the job. A more difficult and unexpected problem was the unpaid time between her appointments with clients:

Much more of a problem than the cost of travel were the gaps between appointments. I could have a 15-minute appointment at, I don't know 7, then another appointment at 9. You couldn't do anything with the time – it was just wasted time and you didn't get paid anything for that time.

Jenny is not alone in highlighting this issue. Unpaid travel time would go on to become the subject of a court case against companies contracted by Haringey Council to provide care services. In that instance, the use of unpaid travel time took down some workers' wages to less than £4 an hour. In Autumn 2020, the workers were awarded £100,000 in back-dated earnings. But even with this precedent, access to the courts is hard for low-paid workers – wins are uncertain, the process drawn out and the innovation in exploitation is often quicker than workers' ability to fight back.

Jenny's stories shocked me most when she talked about being placed in situations for which she had nothing like the knowledge, support, or training to handle. In one case, thanks to staff shortages, Jenny was asked to provide support for a person with dementia. She had never met the client, and had not been scheduled for the appointment at the beginning of the day:

I was asked to cover for a client after somebody had called in sick. The client was a person suffering with dementia. I'd never worked with a dementia patient before, and I'd had no training – I'd been promised it, but it was months away. To top it all off, she didn't speak English and I didn't speak Spanish, so I was left trying to communicate with someone whose language I didn't understand. At points, she got very distressed, and there was nothing I could do to help that – I was also quite distressed [. . .] I ended up being there about four hours.

In the end, on the back of traumatic experiences like this, Jenny left the care sector altogether. Forty per cent of people in social care roles do so every year, leaving the sector with over 100,000 vacancies at any given time.[40]

I felt I was being asked to do things I wasn't qualified to do, and like I'd end up hurting someone. I couldn't take the risk, and it definitely wasn't worth it for the pay and progression.

Jenny's reasons for leaving the sector are consistent with the data on why so many other care workers are leaving their roles.[41] The national body Skills for Care identifies that younger people, people who travel further for work, people on zero-hour contracts, those who do not receive regular training or opportunities to advance qualifications, and those who work in settings with poor standards of care are the most likely groups to leave their roles in any given year. Nearly half leave their job within a year, the majority to work in another sector altogether.[42]

Jenny's story came before Covid. But other social care workers shared their experiences of the pandemic, and how it had impacted them. A senior care manager talked about the fear invading their work life, telling me how:

> Staff are frightened of what could happen. PPE is a concern, and they have gone into isolation after completing an NHS assessment . . . [staff] are frightened to come to work.

Fear, stress and fatigue were common themes. A managing director put things in blunt terms:

> Stress has increased, people are scared. It is likely to get worse. People are physically tired as they have to physically cover others who are self-isolating, many of whom could be at work, but the lack of testing means they have to isolate. The lack of PPE is horrific. Lambs to the slaughter.

I heard the same message from almost every tier of the social care workforce. They had been forgotten. Protective equipment wasn't coming; stress was becoming more unmanageable; and they feared for their safety. A registered manager said:

> The government need to do more with regard to support with PPE, most especially hand sanitizer that is out of reach for most providers. We need more support with aprons, gloves, wet goggles and facemasks.

While a home carer told me:

> [I have] concerns over whether PPE is effective. It's difficult to concentrate. I feel emotional and drained whilst trying to stay positive for clients. I feel it's going to get worse.

'Lambs to the slaughter' is a line that, to me, now reads as tragically prophetic. It is indicative of what a sector run with the twin aims of maximum profit and lowest possible state spend, means for its workers.

THE NATIONAL CARE SERVICE

In the late 1990s and early 2000s, the election of a Labour government raised expectations of bold social care reform. Within the first year of Tony Blair's premiership a royal commission was established – chaired by Sir Stuart Sutherland – to explore how social care was run and funded.

The commission reported just over a year later, and recommended free personal care, based on need and funded by general taxation and a more generous means testing of people to fund their living costs and accommodation.[43] Their recommendations were rejected. The government decided free care would be prohibitively expensive.[44] And while they did adjust the means test for social care living and accommodation costs, it only changed in line with inflation – meaning it did not really become more substantial.

When Blair left office, there was widespread disappointment with his record on social care. Jon Glasby of the University of Birmingham called it a 'tale of policy neglect'. Andrea Rowe, the former chief executive of Skills for Care, said that 'Social care under Blair's leadership has continued to be a 'Cinderella service'. And Bob Hudson, at the University of Durham, noted that it seemed that only health (rather than care) mattered politically.[45]

In 2019, the Labour Party outlined plans to rectify this missed opportunity for lasting change. At their Autumn party conference, and ahead of a December election, they pledged to deliver a National Care Service (NCS) – based on free personal care, better standards for workers and a tougher time for large profit-driven providers. The NCS is now the basis for a current leftist consensus. It has support from academics like Allyson M. Pollock, Luke Clements and Louisa Harding Edgar;[46] trade unions like Unite and GMB;[47] and influential campaign groups like We Own It.[48] Ahead of the 2021 Holyrood elections, the Scottish National Party also committed to delivering a NCS – with SNP leader Nicola Sturgeon calling it a 'top priority' for the Scottish government.[49]

If we take the policies in turn, we find some excellent ideas. Free personal care, the headline proposal in England (implemented in

Scotland in 2002), clearly has merit. Most importantly, it provides a robust delivery mechanism for social care – based on the NHS' own popular principle of 'free at the point of delivery, based on need'. In turn, it immediately addresses variation in care, providing a clear and equal entitlement to social care provision. And while not a policy aimed directly at care costs, it would still immediately reduce the number of people facing catastrophic care costs from around 140,000 people to around 80,000 people.[50]

It is also broadly affordable. It would require spending to increase from around £20 billion per year today, to £36 billion by 2030. That's only £2 billion more per year, in 2030, than the cost of the Conservative Party's 2017 pledge on social care – denigrated as a death tax by *The Daily Mail* and now often cited as a key factor in Theresa May's failure to secure a majority in the 2017 general election.

And it is very popular. YouGov polling in 2018 found that almost three in four English adults support free personal care for all who need it, and that almost 70 per cent would be willing to pay more tax to fund it.[51] Other studies have shown strong cross-party consensus for free personal care, with majority support among both Labour and Conservative voters.[52] Of all the major proposals for social care funding reform, it is by far the easiest to explain – helping it generate its popular appeal.

In terms of the other components of the 2019 Labour manifesto, a better deal for social care workers is clearly important, too. The most common idea is a wage guarantee for care workers. If subsidised by government directly, this could achieve better pay for half a million people – doing highly skilled and intense work – at a cost of £1 billion per year.[53] Other proposals to ensure social care workers have access to development, training and progression are equally vital, in the face of the stories of low hope and exploitation I have already detailed above.

A tougher stance on the worst private providers also makes sense. The Labour Party's 2019 vision for a National Care Service suggests a focus on transparency, financial sustainability and tax compliance. As well as a striking back against private equity, and support sector stability, this would help to address what the Centre for Health and the Public Interest has called 'leakage'. Their research estimates that £1.5 billion of the £15 billion spent on independent care sector 'leaks' out the sector in the form of profit before tax, rent payments, director pay and loan repayments.[54]

THE LIMITS OF THE NCS

The benefits promised by an NCS are undermined by problems that stop it being truly transformational. As a policy around which the left has coalesced, it still needs to be taken further.

Specifically, the National Care Service only asks and answers two of three vitally important questions. The two it answers very well are these: how should better, more accessible care be funded? And by whom? However, to at least some extent, it misses an even more important one: what do we want care to look like? This oversight detaches proposals for a NCS from the lived experiences, needs and ambitions of those who use the social care system.[55]

In *Madness and Civilization*, Michel Foucault explores the evolution of madness.[56] He provides a genealogy of the transition from a time when it was seen as an expression of divinity, something to be treated with kindness, or something that shows the truth of humanity – to a time when it became something that created fear and demanded confinement. His research reveals what he dubs 'the Great confinement' – whereby across Europe, 'insane' people were first segregated to the margins of society, and then segregated physically in medicalised spaces: culminating with the rise of the asylums. He shows how this relates to a wider process of institutionalisation and the enactment of state power, which first defined madness as a moral failure and then as a medical one.

The evolution of social care in the twenty-first century is a modern repetition of the 'great confinement'. On this occasion, the basis is not the binary of mad/sane, but rather vulnerable/normal. From this (false) binary has evolved a highly institutionalised and paternalistic care system designed around the twin goals of i) managing needs and ii) hiding 'vulnerability' from wider society. Predictably, the care system this regime has brought into being is the modern equivalent of the asylum – at least in terms of the power relationship that obtains between the institution and the recipients of care.

This comparison can be shored up through examining how care homes and care at home schemes tend to operate. Too often, care at home functions through the instrument of the 'checklist'. That is, people's 'needs' are boiled down to a mechanical list of the daily chores they need help with. Their support becomes little more than a process of checking off these mechanical chores each day. People become defined, for those who provide their care, not by their humanity, their priorities, their relationships, the life they want to lead and the potential they could reach – but through an oversimplified care plan, that only incidentally relates to what they need. It is a case of need being managed and hidden, rather than actually being met.

One of the worst examples of this one-size-fits-all approach is the continued prevalence of 15-minute appointments. According to Freedom of Information request figures, released by disability charity Leonard Cheshire in 2018, 20,000 people receive visits from their carers that only last 15 minutes.[57] As the charity themselves said, in reacting to these numbers, this can leave a person feeling dismissed and stressed. Reviews have found levels of loneliness in care homes as high as 42 per cent.[58]

Confinement in this system is not about locked doors and padded rooms. Rather, it is a simple result of viewing people through the prism of mechanical tasks, rather than as humans and citizens. More than half of social care users reported feeling isolated in 2017 data.[59] This is a result of a system that views people as problems to be managed, rather than citizens that can be empowered by brilliant public services.

The equivalent of this trend within residential care is 'warehousing'. The modern rise of big, faceless providers has created a system of woefully inadequate care 'factories'. Within these, people often find themselves living lives of idleness, boredom and neglect. In the worst cases, they're packed into small bedrooms – without space for visitors, without scope for even small amounts of autonomy and without design features conductive to social interaction. I have heard care home providers talk about supporting people to do their own laundry as an empowering innovation, in a damning indictment of the extent of our national ambition.

Faced with these modern asylums, the ideas currently mainstreamed within the National Care Service would: help reduce the number of people who lose all their wealth to access this system; help reduce the number of people with no support at all; and would probably bring about some improvements in 'outcomes'. But they do not really change what type of care is provided, what kind of lives it enables and what societal purpose it serves. That is, the NCS does not sufficiently change the nature of care, the power relationships that define it, or the level to which institutionalised and paternalistic care dominates provision.

The experience of Scotland – which has already implemented free personal care (2002) and has a government commitment to a National Care Service (as of 2021) – provides a warning that we still need to develop our ideas, if they are to deliver truly radical change. Survey research by the charity Independent Age shows that, despite almost two decades of free personal care in Scotland, care provision remains inadequate, with 43 per cent of respondents indicating that they did not feel the amount of care they or their family member received was adequate for their needs.[60] The same research also showed how limited the definition of 'free personal care' could be – it covered washing, getting out of bed, meal prep and toileting, but was not perceived to cover shopping, travelling, or support for relationships and social interaction.[61]

THE RIGHT TO A BRILLIANT LIFE

The idea of a service free at the point of delivery, based on need and available to everyone is important, and makes the concept of a National Care Service worth keeping. But it needs to be combined with a stronger vision of what *good care* looks like – that is, what it would deliver, and not just how it would be delivered.

In thinking through the policy implications, the best starting points are the demands that have been developed by those who use social care support – including the disability rights movement. Too often, these are voices left out of social care discourse and debate. The result is policy that, like the NCS, is half formed.

Social Care Future is one organisation with a shared commitment to major transformation in social care – based on focusing less on *who* provides care, and more on *what* care is available and for what *ends*. In June 2019, the group brought together 80 contributors to draft a shared vision in answer to these questions. The first attempt at capturing the vision read:

> We all want to live in the place we call home with the people and things that we love, in communities where we look out for one another, doing the things that matter to us and we're good at. We all want the peace of mind that should we, our families, or neighbours need some support from public services to do so, that it will be there for us quickly and affordably.

> Great support offered, how we want and need it, revives our sense of hope and purpose. It helps all of us keep or regain control over our lives, connect and sometimes reconnect with the things that are most important to us and to realise our potential. By doing so, it allows us

to keep on contributing to our communities, with the benefits rippling out to everyone.

By investing together, we can create a fair, reliable and effective social care support for everyone. By investing in a better social care future, we can invest in us.[62]

Their vision is brilliant because it doesn't ask 'how to make the asylum cheaper, free or state-run' – but rather, how to smash the asylum completely, and move care onto a more empowering, dignified foundation.

Elsewhere, more ambitious conceptions of what care does and achieves have come from within the disabled people's rights movement. In 2019, the Reclaiming Our Futures Alliance of disabled people and disabled people's organisations set out a plan for a National Independent Living Support Service. This detailed a vision for independent living defined not as disabled people doing everything on their own, but rather having choice and control over their lives; being included in the community; and having the same chances to take part as other people.[63] Critically, while it has important overlaps with the NCS, it also calls for more fundamental and ambitious reforms to how social care support works, and what it looks to achieve.

Looking across the deliberative research, there are three changes that need to be better integrated into any conception of, or narrative around, a National Care Service:

1. **Towards Community:** Everyone should have a right to care in their own home and community wherever possible, delivering alongside people they know and places they call home.
2. **Towards Personalisation:** Care should be personalised around an objective to give everyone a brilliant life, rather than being mechanical and one-size-fits-all.
3. **Towards Empowerment:** Care should be undertaken *with* people, not *to* them – with a fundamental recalibration of power between providers, carers, care workers and people receiving support.

If integrated into a future NCS, these changes would combine to form a positive approach to care funding with a more empowering envision of what care looks like and can achieve.

TOWARDS COMMUNITY

The case for delivering more care in the community is well developed. It is in line with what people who use social care services want. It is an excellent way to maintain people's independence and dignity. It avoids people having to pay catastrophic residential costs, as is the norm in care homes.

Despite these prospective benefits, there has been little real progress in bringing more care into the community. A community-led model of care relies on a system that provides support as soon as its needed, with the ambition of maintaining someone's quality of life and capacity to flourish for as long as possible. But severe funding pressures on local authorities have instead left us with a care system that only intervenes at the latest possible moment – often once someone's needs have deteriorated and where intensive support is the only available option.

This can be seen in the international data. The UK has a much higher proportion of people receiving care in residential and nursing homes – and hospitals – than many other, comparable countries.

Table 4.1   Location of Deaths, Selected European Countries and the UK[64]

	Home	Hospital	Care home
European average	33%	44%	18%
UK	23%	47%	28%
Difference	–10%	+3%	+10%

One third of people in Europe can expect to die in their home, compared to just a quarter of people in the UK – despite people overwhelmingly saying that dying at home, surrounded by loved ones, would be their preference. This is one, indicative example of how the UK care system is designed around acute need, late intervention and managing need rather than ensuring dignity, independence, or flourishing lives.

In fact, the situation is highly variable across the UK. In Summer 2021, analysis by the IPPR and CF – a healthcare management consultancy and analysis company – revealed a stark postcode lottery determining who has access to community care. In some local authorities, the best being Hammersmith and Fulham, more than eight in ten people receiving care support were receiving it at home. In others, the figure was less than half – such as just 46 per cent of people in Barnsley.[65]

Some of this can be put down to demographics – the average age of some places is very different to others in the UK. But the variation even exists once local authorities are grouped by geographic and demographic features. Indeed, even a moderately ambitious attempt to close avoidable variation between similar places would help 80,000 people to receive more appropriate care and generate efficiencies worth over £2.5 billion a year.

Everyone should have the opportunity to receive good support, as soon as they need it – and for that care to be in their community and home by default.

TOWARDS PERSONALISATION

Guaranteeing people care at home, from the point they need it, should be an opportunity to focus on personalised rather than one-size-fits-all models. This would mean commissioning significantly more diverse, relational and personalised social care – rather than the mechanical and institutional 'life and limb' services that too often dominate.

Isolated care 'warehouses' and 15 minutes 'flying visits' by over-stretched and underpaid care workers need not be the norm. Models of care do exist that provide people with more choices – or which better tailor care to the needs and demands of a specific diagnosis (e.g., dementia). Indeed, there are many examples of care models that are not used as widely as they could be in this country, but which highlight opportunities for greater personalisation and choice within community care.

There are 150 Shared Lives schemes in the UK. Shared Lives provide opportunities for adults to live, independently, in their community – with the support of a community network. Within the schemes, Shared Lives carers use their own home and family life, to share it with someone who needs support. Carers earn up to £32,500 per year – and receive training, breaks and a support network. It provides a community-based and relationship focused alternative to residential care.

Evaluations of shared living schemes have been positive. Over 96 per cent of Shared Lives schemes are rated good or outstanding across England, compared to just 65 per cent of large independent nursing homes and 72 per cent of large independent care homes.[66] In 2018, an independent review found that Shared Lives can provide a preferable model of respite services for older people and people living with dementia.[67] Moreover, estimates suggest that Shared Lives could offer

£225million of savings per year, if every area caught up to the best performing – thanks to reductions in A&E and hospital admissions.

Buurtzorg is another example of excellent community care, pioneered in the Netherlands. Buurtzorg translates to 'neighbourhood care' and is an innovative homecare model developed in the Netherlands. It is a system designed to allow people with care needs to live independently, with less dependence on formal support.

The model runs as follows. A district nurse provides coaching for the individual and their family, to build their capacity and confidence to deliver care. The focus is on relationships, with nurses encouraged to spend most of their time with people.

Evaluations have suggested the scheme comes with significant benefits. The cost per hour is more expensive. However, the care provided is much higher quality and orientated towards prevention, meaning only half as much care as is needed on average. People live better, more independent lives – in the place they call home, and with people they know – for 40 per cent less cost than traditional homecare models.

In residential settings, where they are needed, fantastically better care could also be within reach. In the village of Hogewey, just outside Amsterdam is one example of a cutting-edge care facility. Hogewey provides a space for around 152 residents, all with advanced dementia, to lead a normal life. The village has a town square, a supermarket, a hairdressers, theatre, pub and restaurant. Living arrangements are designed around familiarity – with different living areas themed. The logic of Hogeway is simple – living a normal life is much easier in a place people can call home, with tailored support, than it is when receiving a very poor level of unspecialised care in a place you no longer recognise. Moreover, in Holland, it is publicly funded through the country's social security system and costs the state no more than other forms of nursing home in the Netherlands, as of 2019.[68]

Research on dementia villages specifically remains nascent, and it can be hard to obtain reliable gauges of quality of life from residents with a dementia diagnosis. But the studies that do exist are encouraging. Reviews have found the higher staffing levels, increased physical activity[69] and a reduction in the use of antipsychotic medication. Before the village was introduced, 50 per cent of residents needed antipsychotic medication, which has since been reduced to 12 per cent of residents (as of 2019).[70] Studies of similar models, like the Eden Alternative in Texas, found a reduction in pressure ulcers, use of restraint, staff absenteeism and an increase in residents' levels of movement – all highly positive indicators for people living with an advanced dementia diagnosis.[71]

It works because it looks to provide people who use it a place and a community that they can call home.

TOWARDS EMPOWERMENT

The market has provided a very paternalistic model of social care in the UK. The status quo today is that care is 'done to people' rather than with them. However, though they have merits, progressive alternatives have rarely put forward ideas that would genuinely change this power dynamic. Indeed, concepts like a National Care Service would arguably reiterate it.

This is not, however, inevitable. There is growing evidence that some ownership models support more equal power relations. Specifically, models of democratic and local ownership – normally using highly innovative approaches, and delivering care at a smaller scale – that are exciting prospects in social care delivery. There is a growing consensus on a definition for 'democratic and local ownership'. In 2020, the New Economics Foundation – themselves, building on work by Co-operatives UK, the University of Manchester and the Centre for Health and the Public Interest – laid out some simple criteria for what democratic, local ownership looks like in practice:

- Legal binding to a clear social mission
- Accountable to people needing and providing support
- Organised at the smallest appropriate scale[72]

If care organisations displaying these values became dominant, it would constitute a major empowerment of people who receive care and of workers who provide care.

There are some excellent examples of emerging, empowering and democratic care provision. For example, there is much that is innovative about Equal Care co-operative, operating in West Yorkshire's Calder Valley. It is a platform co-op, meaning it uses a digital platform to provide its service. Their collaborative platform allows each person to choose their relationships, and then decide where and how their support takes place. It is funded by the community, rather than by private equity, through a community shares model. This model allows investment in enterprises that benefit a community and investors to then have a democratic say. They have proven themselves a remarkably successful form of capital since 2009. And they are multi-stakeholder in design, which means they are governed through dialogue – in this case, with both the providers and recipients of care held in focus.

These are emerging services, with evaluations pending. But the early indications are very strong. Testimony from people using the care service suggests a sense of ownership and empowerment, not always associated with social care. Ambitions include a target to pay new care workers £20,000 per year at the very least – a full 25 per cent above the average in the industry.[73]

There are three main advantages to Equal Care's model. First, its innovative platform allows it to make significant efficiencies. Second, its democratic ownership model allows those efficiencies to be invested in people and workers. Finally, its platform is designed around empowering those members, care recipients and providers alike – helping address problems with power dynamics that often plague other provider models.

Elsewhere, there are promising examples of social enterprises. PossAbilities is one such case, in Greater Manchester. It has been set up to help people live the life they choose, rather than one imposed on them. It provides self-contained living spaces, has a voluntary commitment to the Driving Up Quality code, exclusively 'good' and 'outstanding' ratings from the inspector, its own 'Happiness Manifesto' and a clear space for families and shared lives. These are features of quality and personalisation that are far from standard in this country's care provision.

The wider evidence of democratic and local ownership models in social care specifically is still inchoate, but promising. Equally promising is the extensive evidence on the link between organisations focused on social value and the quality of service provision. Compared to other forms of ownership, co-operative models are associated with greater job satisfaction, worker wellbeing, lower pay inequality and higher rates of engagement and productivity.[74] Despite this, the UK has disproportionately fewer co-operatives and mutuals than other OECD countries (and four times fewer than Germany).[75]

MAKING THE CHANGE

There are clear routes to achieving these three aims – more community, more empowerment and more personalisation – through ambitious new policies. Each are compatible with the National Care Service model. Combined, they provide both a model for delivery (free at the point of need, as in the NHS), and a model for what is delivered (the best possible care).

First, we need a formal guarantee that everyone can have access to care at home, where they would most benefit from it, and a commitment to bringing in innovative models of care to ensure choice and personalisation – all of which will require investment in community infrastructure. The pandemic has showed that we just don't currently have the capacity, services, or staff to deliver in line with a community-first model of care.

That is not to say there wouldn't be a return. In the medium to long-term, community care is not only a fundamentally better way of delivering care, but also a more efficient one. This is intuitive: community care is all about good principles of prevention and early intervention. It is about maintaining independence and dignity and delaying the point at which someone needs more intensive or acute support. The upfront investment needed by community care would pay itself back, in better lives and better public finances alike.

In thinking about the size of investment needed, we can look internationally for inspiration. In the USA, community care infrastructure forms a vital component of President Joe Biden's post-Covid stimulus fund. His investment will equal $400 billion over eight years – or $50 billion per year from his $3 trillion investment package. In the UK the equivalent amount of investment would be worth around £5 billion per year, over the same eight-year period.

This figure would provide the capacity to do two things. First, it would allow community capacity to increase. Research has indicated a £2 billion per year stimulus for community capacity would be a reasonable post-Covid settlement. The remaining money could be invested in a new, social care transformation fund – providing local authorities with the money they need to incubate, scale and transition to community-led, democratically-owned and social anchored care provision.

This extra funding would give the government an opportunity to set ambitious standards for ethics within the social care sector. It has previously been suggested that the government should introduce a binding set of ethical standards for the sector, including:[76]

- A commitment to high quality care: Contracts should only be awarded where there is confidence in quality and where there is a clear accountability mechanism between providers, social care workers, carers and people using support.

- Workforce standards: Contracts should only be awarded where organisations pay a real living wage, provide adequate training and support, and engage in sectoral bargaining.
- Economy: Preference should be given to local organisations, that can demonstrate value to their local economy.
- Environment: Preference should be given to organisations that can provide evidence of high environmental standards.

To this list, we might suggest additions, based on the content of this chapter so far. Firstly, that there should be a set preference for co-operatives, social enterprises, small social care providers – and other promising, empowering models of ownership and delivery. This preference already exists in Wales, where the 2014 Social Services and Wellbeing Act embedded an expectation that these types of social value-focused providers be preferred when commissioning government services.

This could be taken a step further. To accelerate the sustainable transition from large, private equity funded and corporate social care providers, a new expectation could be implemented by stipulating that local authorities spend a set proportion of their commissioning budget on a) small providers embedded in the community, b) direct provision of care by the authority itself, or c) care provided by co-operatives, social enterprises, mutuals, or similar.

Second, there should be a focus on empowerment within these standards. Providers delivering government services should be required to put in place meaningful consultation with care recipients, carers and workers – and to action their views. Their ability to do so should be measured by the satisfaction of people using their services, and the number and type of complaints received about their provision. Any sign of a lack of accountability to the people using these services should be considered a break of contract, and reason enough for a local authority to change providers.

Next, we must recognise that the ongoing crisis experienced by the social care workforce severely limits the potential for transformation. Workers need the security, tools and training to provide great care – and if we do not do right by them, as presently, they cannot do right by us.

The Labour 2019 proposals for an NCS included a pay rise for workers. But we also need mechanisms for more fundamental change – to better train and professionalise care workers, to make it an attractive career going forward and to ensure there is scope for progression – including into roles with autonomy and professional expertise, as we might find in the nursing and medical professions.

There are several ways this could be achieved. Significant investment in training is an obvious one. The national body Skills for Care estimates that 48 per cent of workers in the social care sector do not have a care qualification.[77] Given the kind of high-pressure people in these roles, like Jenny, are under – this lack of provision for training is alarming. It reflects a government that invests a woefully small amount in social care training overall, and in continuing development for professionals more widely.

Perhaps most important is the sector's ability to negotiate collectively. The health sector is full of infrastructure to collectively negotiate, campaign and advocate for different parts of the workforce. There are bespoke unions, like the British Medical Association; there are an array of Royal Colleges; there is a formal infrastructure for formal negotiation on pay, training and recruitment between representatives of the sector and the government. The same cannot be said of social care. If we really want to evolve social care, we need a body to advocate for the evolution of the social care career. This means embedding sectoral and collective bargaining for workers – through something akin to a Royal College of Social Care Workers, with union status.

While the conditions and levels of exploitation experienced by the social care workforce demands immediate attention, this is not the only workforce challenge. Local authorities have also seen huge cuts in their workforce in recent years. In 1999, local government had a headcount of just over 2.7 million employees and central government of 2.3 million. Today, local government has around 2 million employees and central government 3.1 million – a big centralisation of capacity.[78]

One area where expertise has been particularly lost to local authorities is commissioning. The staff with relationships to prospective local providers, and who can differentiate between unscrupulous providers out to make a quick buck and those who would genuinely provide good care, have been lost.[79] Restoring this expertise is vital if we have any hope of local authorities being able to identify, partner with and sustain the kinds of social care providers who can challenge the unaccountability, one-size-fits-all provision, profiteering and paternalism of care as it currently exists.

A BETTER DEAL FOR CARERS

There is one more issue that needs close consideration – the role and work of informal or unpaid carers. One of the tragedies of the initial welfare state, as proposed by Beveridge and enacted by the 1940s Attlee government, was that it simply took for granted unpaid labour.

This was often particularly bad news for women. Indeed, Beveridge's recommendations referred explicitly to the duty of women to marry and provide the labour of social reproduction. Subsequently, his recommendations did not include any state intervention where unpaid labour, often by women, could be relied upon.

As we reimagine health and care, we must not make the same mistake. But it's a risk the National Care Service concept currently runs. In thinking exclusively about the formal social care system, it might be accused of having far too little to say about the informal care being provided outside it.

Before the Covid-19 pandemic, the amount of adult care being provided through informal, unpaid means – rather than through the state – was significant. Official estimates in 2016 put it at 7.9 billion hours a year, from just over 2 million carers.[80] It is thought it would take 4 million adult social care workers, working every week of the year at their median hours, to replace those providing informal care.

The consequences of providing large amounts of care, without the proper levels of support, can be severe. Providing unpaid care alongside work can be particularly difficult – with new estimates of the number juggling work and care much higher than once thought, at 4.87 million.[81] 2.6 million people gave up work to care during 2019, and 2 million reduced their working hours to facilitate unpaid care.[82] This underpins a strong association with poverty. Research by the New Policy Institute found that among people providing 20 hours or more of care each week, 37 per cent are living in poverty – compared to one in five people in the whole population.[83] High levels of unpaid care are a significant driver of gender inequality, with estimates suggesting women provide 60 per cent more unpaid care than men overall.

There are several trends that suggest the burden of unpaid care on people's lives will increase significantly in the future. The number of older people receiving informal care is predicted to increase by 60 per cent on 2010 levels, by 2030.[84] As the population ages, the average age of an unpaid carer is also likely to increase. Around 60 per cent of informal adult care is already provided by people older than 60, and that figure is increasing – meaning a situation where many could simultaneously have their own support needs and be providing care to someone else.

Covid-19 is a case study in how unprepared we are for rising demands on unpaid care and informal carers. There is clear evidence that care-givers experienced a significant burden during the pandemic.[85] In many cases, this was down to higher needs of the care recipient, the loss of support services, a lack of opportunities for rest and respite and increased hours of care – all of which could become business as usual in the future, even without another pandemic taking place.[86]

While there are lots of areas where more support can be introduced – and would be both welcome and impactful – the key concern for carers today is often financial support. At present, Carers Allowance is a paltry sum at just over £60 per week. This lack of financial support not only leaves carers vulnerable, but incentivises government to neglect funding improvements in the social care system, because unpaid labour can be cheaply relied upon.

According to the Office for National Statistics, unpaid carers provided social care worth £59 billion a year in 2014, representing an almost 50 per cent rise from just 2005.[87] This figure means, ultimately, that it could cost as much as this to replace unpaid carers with paid carers. On the current trajectory, it may be that this becomes inevitable. However, the better and more proactive policy would include providing unpaid carers with a significant dividend for their contribution.

For example, a care benefit-share scheme, which allocated carers 25 per cent of the economic value they create – just for adult care – would cost around £15 billion a year. That would equate to a payment worth £7,500 for every recipient of care, to support the people providing their care – a figure twice as high as the current Carers Allowance benefit. Importantly, this higher level of payment would better encourage direct state provision of care in the future – whereas free care currently incentivises them to avoid increasing care provision.

There is extensive international evidence showing that a much fairer deal between state and carers is both possible and effective. In Germany, cash payments are offered to carers – either to purchase services or support their carers – with payments ranging from £3,500 to £21,000 per year. Evaluations suggest this is more cost effective and more popular than the care home-led and highly institutionalised model currently offered in England. Importantly, the payment suggested here would be delivered alongside state services – as support for unpaid carers, rather than a personal care budget.

Elsewhere, there are other international examples of support for carers that the UK would do well to adopt. For instance, the UK lags behind on compassionate leave policies, providing no specific entitlement to even unpaid leave. In Poland, carers are entitled to two days paid leave per year worked, with financial entitlement based on 80 per cent of average earnings (essentially, a carers furlough).[88] Adopting this scheme would be straightforward, given the infrastructure developed during the pandemic, and would provide much needed space for individuals to grieve. Furthermore, in supporting people to remain in work, it would come with its own gains. Carers UK estimated in 2013 that supporting carers to stay in work, through policies like this, could add as much as £5.3 billion to the UK economy.[89]

Our society needs carers, and the vision should not be to replace them entirely. But what is certain is that the state cannot, sustainably, go into the future taking carers for granted. It must invest in their wellbeing, share the value of their care and pick up its fair share through the social care system.

5

The Sustainability Frontier

The UK was meant to be world leading when it came to major health shocks. In the Global Health Security Index's (GSHI's) 2019 assessment of our capacity to respond to a disease outbreak, we were ranked second – only behind the United States.[1] By Spring 2021, the UK and the United States ranked first and fifth respectively for total Covid-19 deaths – and both were in the top 15 globally, when ranked by deaths per 100,000 people.[2] The countries ranked bottom and second from bottom in the GHSI's 2019 table – Turkey and Albania – had both fared markedly better.[3]

It might seem logical to think that this experience will change how we approach health resilience and sustainability. But, in fact, there is a very real risk that we learn entirely the wrong lessons and repeat our past mistakes. There are pitfalls for both the left and the right, which threaten to undermine our ability to translate the experience of Covid-19 into a UK policy that adds to – rather than detracts from – global health sustainability.

One blind alleyway is an emerging deployment of a 'health security' paradigm, including by the Tory government. In the Spring of 2021, they announced a new body designed to deal with infectious disease threats. Originally, this was to be called the National Institute for Health Protection. At the last minute the name was changed, in favour of 'Health Security Agency'.[4] The deadline-day change indicates an intentional shift in emphasis.

Of course, this emphasis is about more than just the names of new Whitehall departments. In one of his first speeches on the post-Covid future, entitled 'Reinvigorating our System for International Health', former Secretary of State for Health and Social Care Matt Hancock said:

> The pandemic has thrust the G7 health agenda to the centre of global affairs. Health policy is the number one economic policy, security policy. Today I want to set out the UK's G7 agenda for the rest of this

year and also some of the actions we're putting in place immediately to deliver on it. The first area is health security – for everyone.[5]

Whether or not it is couched in the language of equality, 'security' is a loaded concept. Rather than looking to identify, understand and solve the structural reasons for the growing global risk from infectious diseases, it implies a focus on borders and control. It denotes less effort to prevent pandemics and major disease outbreaks elsewhere, and greater efforts to insulate the UK and its borders – so we can avoid the damage when such diseases do emerge. In essence, security is a paradigm that allows rich countries to continue concentrating resource in places where the risk of diseases emerging and doing significant damage are lowest. It is therefore, often, a nativist approach to global health.

And while it's framed as a break from the policies that made the UK and the world so vulnerable to a pandemic, it can in fact be seen as a reiteration or deepening of the pre-pandemic policy status quo. Research by Kate Jones of London's Institute of Zoology has shown a rise in emerging diseases, concentrated on new disease 'hotspots' (areas where conditions are right for disease emergence) in parts of the world with lower latitudes.[6] That is, the risk of infectious disease outbreaks before Covid-19 were concentrated in places where public health capacity and investment is lowest, and reporting is weakest. Jones concludes that 'global resources to counter disease emergence are poorly allocated'.[7] The countries with the best early warning systems and surveillance approaches are not the same as those facing the greatest risks.

That is the status quo that an undue focus on security could further entrench. For instance, one worrying indicator in the aftermath of Covid-19 has been a focus in many advanced economies in the West on developing domestic vaccine manufacturing capacity. They have realised the value to self-interest of the ability to hoard vaccines produced at home – an approach that is hugely damaging at a global scale. At the time of writing, the UK government has been clear its ambition is to attract more manufacturing capability from elsewhere.[8]

Nativism is unlikely to be an optimal approach in a world defined by vulnerability to chronic and infectious diseases. In Covid-19, we have proof that a nationalistic and isolationist security agenda is no match for the level of vulnerability a highly interconnected and inter-reliant global health system faces. Focusing on national security in the face of pandemics when they strike, rather than addressing the fundamental reasons we have become so vulnerable to emerging diseases, is entirely the wrong path.

It's not, however, only the current government and the political right who risk learning the wrong lessons from Covid-19. In the aftermath of the pandemic, the left is also at risk of defining their asks more narrowly; becoming more inward looking, or otherwise not quite grasping the scale of the health challenge posed by this new 'era of pandemics'.

Specifically, the experience of Covid-19 risks strengthening the kinds of approaches to health I have questioned throughout this book: NHS-centrism and a purely defensive position. It would be little surprise, for example, if the poor performance of outsourcing – by Deloitte, Serco, Sitel and others – leads our movement to focus ever more on who provides NHS services. Undeniably, this is important. But as a sole focus, it simply isn't in proportion to the scale of thinking needed in a world that has experienced the shock of Covid.

It would take another full book – and perhaps several – to properly understand the global health order, and how it needs to change. Some of these books already exist, and provide compelling reasons why the World Health Organisation, existing norms, vaccine and treatment supply chains, health treaties and international health infrastructure aren't anything like fit for purpose. I do not intend to spend a few thousand words oversimplifying their points. Instead, and consistent with this book's search for a blueprint for UK public health, I explore what domestic levers exist to embed sustainability and global solidarity in this country's approach.

GLOBAL HEALTH IS DESTABILISING RAPIDLY

Covid-19 was not only predictable but predicted. Elected decision makers might like to put it down to bad luck or interpret it as a shock once in a lifetime occurrence – a 'black swan' event. But this would be to give in to a comfortable delusion. The truth is Covid-19 is a symptom of a fundamental rise in global health vulnerability and the era of pandemics in which we now live.

Instances of prescience are easy to find. In 2014, a team led by Professor Katherine Smith analysed a novel dataset, covering the period 1980 to 2013. This covered 12,102 outbreaks of 215 human infectious diseases. Even with stringent controls for disease surveillance, communications, geography and host availability, they found a significant rise in the total number and diversity of disease outbreaks. That indicates not only an increasing risk of major disease outbreaks, but that the risk is increasing more quickly than humans are developing capabilities in surveillance, warning and prevention.[9]

It is not just in technical academic journal papers that we find predictions of rising pandemic risk, either. They can also be found in the very places policy makers and politicians look most readily for insight and ideas. In early 2019, a white paper was released through the World Economic Forum, documenting the results of a new study on World Health Organisation global outbreak data.[10] It showed how the risk of global disease outbreaks had steadily dropped in the late twentieth century. Alarmingly, it also showed how that progress had been reversed in just the last decade. In the twenty years before 2010, the number of countries experiencing 'significant disease outbreaks' halved – from 36 to 18. Between 2010 and 2018, the number more than doubled, from 18 to 37. It is a trend towards exponential growth in infectious disease events with pandemic potential.[11]

Penning the foreword, Peter Sands – research fellow at Harvard's Global Health Institute and former CEO of Standard Chartered – showed his own foresight:

> Neurobiologically conditioned, as we are, to pay attention to stark contrasts and sudden changes, we often overlook slow moving changes in our environments that may herald disastrous consequences. The evolution of infectious disease risk is one such change. As this report explains, the number and diversity of infectious disease outbreaks are gradually but inexorably increasing, as is their capacity to send shocks through our global economic systems. As we travel, trade and communicate across an increasingly hyperconnected global economy, more and more companies will find themselves exposed to the effects of outbreaks that begin thousands of miles away.[12]

As Sands indicates, we had not got to grips with the risk. But we cannot pretend there were not warning shots before Covid-19 – including SARS, swine flu, avian flu and zika virus. A major health shock was very much on the cards, and that means we must contend with Covid as symptomatic of a chronic trend, rather than an acute crisis.

That means recognising and reacting to the fact that the risk of pandemics in the future are not less likely because of Covid. It would be easy to commit a gambler's fallacy: to believe that because an event has happened in the recent past, it is less likely to happen again soon. But unless both domestic and global policy changes, Covid-19 by itself does nothing to reduce the odds of further major health shocks.

As much as we should worry about the increase in frequency of global disease outbreaks, we should also worry about the prospect of an emerging infectious disease that is more infectious or deadly than Covid-19. The World Health Organisation's list of 'top emerging diseases likely to cause major epidemics' contains some lethal prospects:

Table 5.1   Description of a Sample of EIDs of Significant Concern

Name of Emerging Disease	Description/Symptoms	Comparison to Covid-19
Crimean Congo Haemorrhagic Fever	A viral disease that can cause fever, muscle pains, headache, vomiting, diarrhoea, bleeding, liver failure and death	Case fatality rate of up to 40 per cent[13]
Ebola Virus Disease	A viral disease that can cause fever, weakness, rash, reduced kidney and liver function and death	Case fatality rate of 25 to 90 per cent[14]
Marburg Virus Disease	From the same family as Ebola, causing severe headache, malaise, high fever and rapid debilitation	Case fatality rate of between 24 and 88 per cent[15]
Lassa Fever	Can cause fever, tiredness, weakness, headaches, bleeding gums, vomiting or low blood pressure	Case fatality rate of 1 per cent, rising to 15 per cent for patients hospitalised with severe cases[16]
Nipah Virus Infection	Can cause fever, headache, drowsiness, disorientation and respiratory issues. May lead to coma within 24–48 hours	Case fatality rate of between 40 and 75 per cent[17]

This is just a small sub-section of infectious diseases of global concern. Notably, highly pathogenic Coronaviruses – a genre containing Covid-19 (SARS-CoV-2) – was also listed as a priority by the World Health Organisation in their 2015 list, indicating that these are not simply distant threats to our health.

Another temper for complacency is the fact that emerging infectious diseases could pose a greater scientific challenge – in terms of producing a vaccine or a cure – than Covid. While violent political apathy delayed the development of effective treatments for HIV/AIDS – itself a case study of an emerging zoonotic disease – the process was further complicated by the biology of the virus. AIDs is a disease that enters the human genome, making a total cure very difficult (though suppression has proven possible).[18] It is a remarkable thing that we ended the first year of the Covid-19 pandemic with viable new treatments and vaccines – albeit with huge challenges around distributing those, but within countries and globally – but there is no guarantee our science will provide an absolute safety net, particularly given how little pre-emptive work there is on emerging infectious diseases.

As well as the lesser-known viruses in *Table 5.1*, influenzas remain a genus of disease with the potential to start a pandemic of significant destructive power. The scale of flu as a threat should not be understated. When it comes to historic disease outbreaks, Spanish Flu (H1N1) is perhaps only less well known than the Black Death and killed somewhere between 50 and 100 million people (c.5 per cent of the global population).[19] In 2009, a strain of H1N1 ('Swine Flu') killed 12,000 people in the United States including over 1,000 children. In the UK, where 392 people died, worst case scenario planning showed potential outcomes where 30 per cent of the UK population were infected and 65,000 people died. Despite this, many struggled to take the risk seriously, with an indicative *Daily Mail* headline from the time reading 'How £300 Million Was Squandered on Swine Flu Jabs that We Didn't Need'.[20] Until now, the right media has been less than favourable on governments who spend money on resilience.

While we are unable to predict the next flu epidemic, we do have a good indication of the biggest risks. Studies note a variety of subtypes of swine and avian-originating flu have high pandemic potential – including some for which the human population currently lacks the antibodies that would provide some degree of resistance.[21]

Elsewhere, the threat is not emerging diseases, but re-emerging illnesses. There are some shocking mechanisms by which we might find ourselves facing diseases otherwise lost to history. Among the most alarming sources of emerging diseases could be the reduction in the Arctic's permafrost. Studies of glacier ice cores have shown active viruses in samples up to 15,000 years old. Some of these viruses are known, whilst some were entirely new to modern science.[22]

It might seem intuitively unlikely that this could lead to outbreaks, but there have already been warnings. A 2016 outbreak of Anthrax in Siberia – which led to the culling of 200,000 reindeer and killed one human – was linked to thawing permafrost.[23] Any individual outbreak linked to permafrost remains unlikely, but it reiterates a worrying point: a huge number of factors are combining to substantially increase the chances, in any given period, of a lethal and disruptive health shock. This is the mechanism of growing global health vulnerability.

THE BOUNDARIES OF GLOBAL PUBLIC HEALTH

I opened this chapter by noting that the UK had come second in the Global Health Security Index. This league table now provides a historical document of the flaws in how we'd defined 'good' when it came to preparedness. Because it wasn't just the UK who scored well in the league tables and then did badly during Covid. A 2020 research paper led by Enoch Abbey, from the Johns Hopkins School of Medicine, found that the Global Health Security Index was not predictive of response or performance in light of the coronavirus outbreak.[24] If this indicates anything, it is most of all how flawed our definitions of 'good' were.

As important as the political failure to recognise the threat pandemics pose has been the failure to develop compelling conceptual frameworks, through which a good approach to global health can be embedded.[25] Accepting that pandemics and disease outbreaks are a chronic risk of the twenty-first century is not enough. We will only come to the right solutions if better able to account for the structural reasons behind rising vulnerability.

Left and grassroots movements have developed compelling concepts and models to better understand and inform action on other existential-level threats. This is particularly true in work around our climate and nature emergency. Kate Raworth has developed the Doughnut model, an alternative to traditional economic figures like supply and demand graphs, with sustainability built in. She builds on earlier work by Rock-ström et al., which established the 'safe operating space for humanity'.[26] Global public health needs a similar framework – a model that understands the domains of risk that moderate our exposure to emerging and re-emerging diseases, around the world. We need to be clear what the limits of tolerance are for global public health, just as our movements are ever clearer on the limits of tolerance for activities that impact planetary health.

Table 5.2   The Safe Operating Space for Humanity, Global Public Health

Global Public Health Boundaries
Climate change
Changing human/animal interaction
Insensitivity of agriculture
Population growth
Urbanisation
Conflict and displacement
Global poverty and inequality
Global trade
Global travel

The challenge of restoring global health sustainability cannot be understated. Nevertheless, there is much here we still have the power to change. Every global health boundary explored above is amenable to policy – but we must act quickly, and we must act decisively.

a. Climate Change

The link between climate warming and emerging infectious diseases has long been evidenced. Through the late 1990s and into the 2000s, research by Jonathan Patz highlighted a link between changing trends in average temperature and both the incidence and distribution of vector-borne diseases.[27] As he even noted then, his conclusions shouldn't be particularly surprising. In fact, humans have had evidence that climatic conditions impact on epidemic infections for centuries.

While the impact of climate variables is never unrelated to modifying influences – levels of poverty, population density, connectivity, farming – there are some clear and worrying trends. Firstly, small changes in temperature can expand the areas in which a pathogen or vector can thrive – or otherwise push them to unprepared geographies. Second, gradual changes in temperature drive evolutionary responses in pathogens and vectors, changing their characteristics. Or slightly warmer environments can increase the incubation period of pathogens, simply making them last longer.

Models have looked to outline the impact of future climate scenarios on infectious diseases. Increasing temperature and precipitation has been linked to increasing malaria transmission in the African highlands.[28] All reasonable models of climate change have been linked to better conditions for malaria transmission in Zimbabwe.[29] Research has come to similar conclusions when looking at arboviruses in south Florida,[30] the West Nile virus,[31] the consequences of El Niño on water-borne diseases in Peru[32] and the transmission of dengue fever.[33] More recent research has linked greenhouse gas emissions and the resulting change in global temperatures, with infectious disease risks linked to ticks, mosquitos, West Nile virus and an increased number of foodborne illnesses.[34]

Against this, the progression of climate warming – driven by the burning of fossil fuels and greenhouse gasses – shows little sign of abating. Between 1990 and 2019, global CO_2 emissions rose by 62 per cent.[35] In 2018, levels of greenhouse gasses in the atmosphere reached a new peak – at 407.8 parts per million.[36] Worryingly, even the break in economic and human activity enforced by Covid-19 did not stop the trajectory of climate change. Global carbon emissions fell by just 6.4 per cent – far below what many researchers had predicted, and in line with a bounce back by 2022.[37] On current trajectories, warming is likely to exceed 3 degrees Celsius – an outcome described as catastrophic in a signed letter from more than 15,000 scientists from 184 countries, published in 2017.[38]

The UK makes a disproportionate contribution to greenhouse gas emissions – meaning we make a disproportionate contribution to our own global health vulnerability. In 2018, the University of Leeds compared UK emissions to sustainable output. They showed that the UK should have 1.6 tonnes of CO_2 emissions per year, per capita, at most; it should use no more than 0.9 kilograms of phosphorous in agricultural soils per year; and it should use no more than 8.9 kilograms of nitrogen from industrial and international biological fixation. Yet, the current performance of the UK is 12.1 tonnes CO_2; 5.2 kilograms of phosphorus and 72.9 kilograms of nitrogen per capita – representing a 756 per cent; 578 per cent and 819 per cent use of allocation respectively.[39]

The impact in global warming is not felt equally across the world. The UK's land temperature is set to increase by less than in many other countries – but this is no cause for relief. In fact, the countries with the highest vulnerability to emerging and re-emerging infectious diseases are often the same as those that will be hit hardest by the impacts of the climate emergency.[40] This means climate emergency could increase vulnerability most in the places where global shock events are almost most likely to originate, amplifying their impact.

b. Human Animal Interaction and Intensive Agriculture

Within the category of emerging and re-emerging infectious diseases, the biggest threat is posed by zoonotic diseases transmitted to humans by animals. As such, one of the clearest risks is increased human encroachment into animal habitats, and the rise in intensive animal-based agriculture. These two factors constitute a bridge through which pathogens transmissible between humans and animals can emerge, evolve and take hold.[41]

The threat of this happening had been observed in practice many times before Covid-19. In 2001, a paper led by Dr Peter Daszak explored several emerging diseases and explored whether anthropogenic actions impacting animal habitats were increasing the risks posed by zoonotic diseases. His results were worrying. Habitat loss helped disease emergence in several cases. For two diseases in the study, it was the prime driver. In the case of the Nipah virus – a disease with a case-fatality rate of between 40 and 75 per cent – intensive farming brought together fruit bats and pigs, enabling transmission from the former to the latter. In 1998, the virus transmitted from pigs to humans, via the pig-farm workers, resulting in the first ever human fatalities from the virus.[42]

Since the early 2000s, the link between agricultural practices and emerging diseases has only become clearer. In 2019, research led by Professor Jason Rohr, of the University of Notre Dame, concluded that agricultural drivers were associated with more than a quarter of all emerging infectious diseases since 1940 – and 50 per cent of all emerging zoonotic infectious diseases.[43] This finding has now been repeated in systematic reviews.[44]

There are several causal mechanisms behind it. Perhaps most obviously, increases in agriculture often lead to increased interaction between human and animals. The trend of encroaching into previously wild land then brings human and livestock into closer contact with wildlife. As Bryony Jones and others put it in a review conducted for the Department of International Development:

[. . .]the interaction of humans or livestock with wildlife exposes them to sylvatic disease cycles and the risk of spill over of potential pathogens. Livestock may become intermediate or amplifier hosts, in which pathogens can evolve and spill over into humans, or humans be infected directly from wildlife vectors.[45]

In other words, our food production practices have put in place the conditions for new infectious diseases to emerge, evolve and spread.

Despite this body of evidence, established over decades, intensive agriculture continues to expand. Today, over half the world's habitable land is used for agriculture.[46] Of that, 77 per cent is used for livestock, and 23 per cent for crops – despite the fact the former makes up only 18 per cent of the world's calories (normally, in the diets of the most affluent).[47]

c. Population Growth and Urbanisation

The 1700s and 1800s saw modest annual rises in the global human population, normally of a few tenths of a per cent. At the start of the eighteenth century, the world's population was 600 million and by the end of the nineteenth it was just short of 2 billion. In the following century, population growth exploded. A combination of rising birth rates and declining mortality saw the population hit 2 billion in 1928 and 5 billion in 1987. 1968 marked 'peak population growth' – with the global population increasing 2.1 per cent that year.

Population growth is expected to continue to rise less quickly in the next century – though, by historical records, it will mostly remain rapid. By 2050, the world's population is expected to hit 9.7 billion, and by 2100, it will be almost 11 billion. At that point, it is likely to plateau, or drop.[48] These numbers come with huge uncertainty. The human impact of war, famine, climate change, medical advance, disease, or government policy could yet disrupt these trends. Nonetheless, planning must take account of the fact that, in all likelihood, the number of humans on Earth will only continue to grow throughout most of our lifetimes.

Population growth provides a predictor of emerging infectious diseases. In general studies, population growth as a variable has been linked to zoonotic EID events.[49] In some ways, there are obvious mechanisms behind this – more humans mean more of the interactions (e.g., with animals) that can lead to a disease outbreak. In other cases, the precise ways the world has changed and adapted to a larger population has created specific and avoidable risks.

While we may have fewer resources at our disposal to address population growth, we do have options about how the world changes as it looks to cope with a larger, total population. For example, the spatial consequences of population growth have both helped drive recent global health vulnerability and offered opportunities to address that vulnerability in the future.

One of the key dimensions has been urbanisation. 2007 marked the first time in history that more people in the world lived in urban rather than rural areas, according to the UN's estimates. By 2050, it is predicted that that figure will increase to two-thirds of the world's population.[50] And while urban areas tend to have higher living standards at an aggregate level – high density living has brought about challenges like over-crowding. Globally, almost one in three people living in an urban area live in a slum.[51]

In some ways, twenty-first century urbanisation has elements that increase the vulnerability of urban spaces (and thus the world) – distinct from processes of urbanisation seen in previous centuries. One paper led by the University of Lincoln's Creighton Connolly concludes that 'Contemporary patterns of extended urbanisation fundamentally shift the vulnerability of cities to infectious diseases in ways that differ from those that have historically been associated with urbanisation'.[52] There are few better conditions for infectious diseases to spread than through high-density, highly connected urban spaces. As is shown through examining the association between urbanisation and the impact of infectious diseases since the turn of the millennium.

d. Global Poverty and Inequality

One of the clearest drivers of emerging and re-emerging infectious diseases is global poverty. In many cases, poverty and inequality underpin the emergence of infectious disease by driving many of the trends discussed in this section already. The combination of poverty and urbanisation can lead to squalid living conditions, where waterborne diseases thrive, evolve and are exposed to new forms of pollution.[53] Poverty has a well-established link to deforestation as well – as people expand into forests and other biospheres to sustain a living.

In 2014, a team led by Almudena Marí Saéz explored the conditions behind the severe Ebola outbreak in West Africa.[54] Their evidence implicated bats in the outbreak – specifically, insectivorous free-tailed bats. Contextually, the authors note that the district that the index case for the outbreak – Meliandou – had been known forest region, but had lost approximately 80 per cent of its trees and most of its vegetation in preceding decades. This, in turn, facilitated the closer living and interaction between people and infected species. The first person infected was a two-year-old child playing in a hollow tree.

As well as supporting the conditions for the emergence or re-emergence of infectious diseases, global poverty and inequality accelerate the spread and exacerbate the impact of pathogens. Poverty cannot be disaggregated from levels of sanitation, close proximity of living and lack of clean water. There is compelling evidence, from Covid-19 and prior outbreaks, that urban centres with higher levels of poverty experience the most brutal impacts and largest infection spikes from infectious disease outbreaks.[55]

While genuine global equality, and an end to all forms of poverty, have of course not been realised – there has been progress. Between 1990 and 2015, the number of people living on less than $1.90 a day decreased from 35 per cent to 10 per cent of the world's population.[56] Decreases have also been observed on higher lines of $3.20 and $5.50 a day.[57] Nonetheless, this progress remains very tenuous. Much of the decrease is attributable to China and India, meaning extreme poverty has become concentrated in certain regions, including sub-Saharan Africa.[58] Equally, many recent gains in extreme poverty stand to be undone by the experience of Covid-19 itself – with the World Bank estimating that as many as a further 150 million people will be pushed into extreme poverty – the first rise since 1998.[59]

e. Global Trade and Travel

One of the remarkable traits of the Black Death was its ability to spread. The first introduction to Europe occurred in the Crimea. By mid-1348, the virus had spread through Italy, East Spain, most of France and Greece. By 1349, major outbreaks had hit England and Germany. By 1350, the spread reached Scotland, Northern Ireland and much of Scandinavia.

For a long time, the common knowledge was that fleas and rats spread the Black Death. More recent experimental data challenges this hypothesis. In 2019, Katharine Dean and her colleagues developed a conceptual model to establish whether rats/flea transmission or human transmission were more likely. They concluded with a strong likelihood that it was in fact human to human transmission that spread and sustained the Black Death.[60]

The reason the Black Death thrived was down to its remarkable biology. Several traits of the virus underpinned its success. Some studies have indicated a very long gestation period – with estimates suggesting more than a month between infection and symptoms.[61] Its infectiousness peaks before a person is symptomatic – making it incredibly hard to contain. Combined with a long incubation period, this made quarantine policies incredibly difficult.

Today, it does not take a virus with simply remarkable biology to wreak havoc. Rampant globalisation means a far wider range of diseases have the capacity to survive and spread across borders, where they wouldn't have been able to do so in most of human history. This is down to the significant increase in cross-border connectivity between people and places – driven by a combination of global trade and travel, resulting from wider globalisation.

Cross-border interactions are far more frequent and diverse than ever before. According to the World Tourism Organisation – part of the United Nations – tourism has increased exponentially. The 1950s saw just tens of millions of international tourism arrivals. By 1970, the figure had risen to nearly 200 million. By 1990, it had more than doubled, to over 400 million. And in 2018, the figure reached a new record: 1.4 billion international arrivals.[62]

We need not just look at global travel, either – global trade is also on the rise. Analysis of trade data from 1800 to 2014 shows global trade rising exponentially to 2008 – before levelling out in the years following the financial crash.[63] Compared to 1913, international trade had grown 40 times larger by 2014.[64] This exponential growth represents a meteoric rise in interactions – whether the infrastructure needed to transport goods (haulage, freight, air transport), or the infrastructure needed to govern such a sprawling trade system (international offices, business travel, government departments). That is, it indicates a more connected world, with ever more intensive cross-border interaction.

The right to movement is, correctly, defended by many within the broad church of progressive thought. The implication here is not that people lose the right to flee prosecution, to travel, or to migrate for economic or other reasons. Instead, we should question the power dynamics that allow the benefits of trade and travel to predominantly accrue to wealthier people and countries, and for those activities to take place beyond what is sustainable for the world.

The right response, then, is for a redirection of the rules that govern travel and trade. As campaigner Kierra Box has put it: 'simply put, trade rules exist to make it easier to trade – and increase the amount of all trade globally. Their primary aim is not to end poverty or lower carbon emissions'.[65] The right response is to reshape national and international rules to make global health sustainability a core part of how trade and travel systems work. That might mean fundamental changes to the World Trade Organisation, giving domestic law primacy over international trade, or raising shared production values. It might mean bringing the concept of a Public Net Zero, discussed in Chapter 3, to bear on activities that harm global health – not just domestic health.

f. Conflict and Displacement

Whilst trade and tourism represent indulgences of commercial globalisation, they are not the only ways that human movement can increase the potency and potential impacts of pandemics. This can also come down to population movement resulting from conflict and displacement.

Refugees constitute a major area of growth in the intercontinental movement of people – whether fleeing war, violent conflict, environmental disaster, or political discrimination. Many elements of the current refugee experience can lend themselves to creating and sustaining outbreaks of infectious diseases, including emerging infectious diseases – notably, malnutrition, overcrowding, unhygienic conditions and a lack of basic medical services. All of which are common in formal refugee camps.[66]

In 2007, a paper in the journal *Emerging Infectious Diseases* superimposed outbreaks of recent emerging or re-emerging infectious disease outbreaks onto countries affected by conflict between 1990 and 2006. The overlap was significant, with sites of significant conflict overlapping with major outbreaks of Ebola, H5N1 influenza, monkeypox, plague and malaria.[67] This included cases where otherwise successful eradication of disease broke down – malaria had been virtually eliminated in Tajikistan in the 1960s – but following civil war in 1992/3, and a huge displacement of people to neighbouring countries, malaria parasites returned in 1994. By 1997, cases hit 30,000 per year.[68]

Problems can range. Conflict often undermines surveillance and early warning systems, meaning public health interventions come too late. People are forced to move, whether as refugees or because conflict and emergency demands a redeployment of people. Healthcare settings are often stretched. Supply chains – for both resources and information – are difficult to maintain. And due to medical shortages, inappropriate and outdated medicines can be used – with poor treatment compliance – supporting the development of drug resistance.[69]

In short, environments that lead to large numbers of refugees also create the conditions for infectious diseases to emerge, spread, or otherwise be reintroduced to places where they'd formerly been eradicated – often with huge human cost. It should not be lost on us, of course, that the Black Death is often thought to have been introduced to Europe during a siege (of Caffa) – while the Spanish flu was amplified, significantly, by the movement of people after World War One.[70]

This should accentuate alarm at the projected increase in refugee populations – driven by the consequences of climate change, global inequality and political tension. One estimate from the Institute for Economics and Peace – a thinktank that produces global terrorism and peace indexes – predicted 1.2 billion people from 31 countries were at risk of displacement from ecological threats alone.[71] By way of comparison, the UN's human rights agency had capacity to resettle just over 60,000 people in 2019.[72]

A HEALTHY WORLD FOR FUTURE GENERATIONS

How can we reflect the implications of this understanding of global health vulnerability in UK health policy?

One of the most important interventions in the aftershock of Covid would be a legal guarantee to protect future generations from the impact of pandemics, and other consequences from growing global health insecurity. As it stands, younger and future generations are not just set to be economically worse off than their parents, they face what has been called a 'toxic inheritance'.[73] This includes climate change, species extinction, destabilised oceans and – now, as the pandemic has proven – the growing plight of infectious diseases.

If it is often noted that children today are to be worse off than their parents economically – then we should also note that we are close to the first generation in the modern medical era that will have worse health than its parents. Research already shows stagnating life expectancy in countries like England – and actively declining life expectancy in the poorest parts of our country.[74]

Worse, many of the drivers of the remarkable health gains seen in the twenty-first century are far from guaranteed into the future. The fact we are exceeding the boundaries of global public health is also driving alarming rates of resistance to anti-microbials, meaning we face going into an uncertain future without anti-biotics and a range of other vital medicines.

The global and national consequences of anti-microbial resistance (AMR) are already plain. Today, 123 countries report extensive multi-drug resistant tuberculosis. Up to 2 billion people lack effective access to antimicrobials globally, and 700,000 die at the hands of drug resistant infections. That figure is predicted to rise to 10 million, with a cumulative cost of $100 trillion, if by 2050 is no action is taken.[75] Like the emerging diseases explored in this chapter so far, AMR is sustained and accelerated by instances where we exceed the boundaries of sustainable global health. Its links to poverty, hunger, irresponsible agricultural practice and climate change are well known.[76]

It is not uncommon to see news articles predicting that we'll reach new heights in human longevity. Scientists can almost guarantee a front page by making bold predictions on how long humans will live in the future. As recently as May 2021, a prediction humans would reach 150 years old made a splash in *The Telegraph*.[77] Various predictions by Dr Aubrey de Grey that the first person to live to 1,000 – or even, that the first immortal child – has already been born have been widely covered.[78]

But in reality, our future is far more uncertain than the steady, linear progress we've become used to in the last seventy years. A combination of health shocks, chronic illness, rising socio-economic inequality and resistant microbes could wipe out decades of health progress. Which is to say that the relatively healthy 100 years we've experienced is at genuine risk of being little more than a remarkable blip in history.

It is vital we protect future generations from the damage to health sustainability we are facing today. One of the best ways of doing this would be the introduction of a Future Generations Act, providing formal legal recognition of the right of people to live in a stable public health environment. The intent would be to embed the kind of health sustainability definitions outlined here – which are significantly preferable to the limited definitions of 'security' that ranked the UK second on global health in 2019 – and to shift the UK's culture of policymaking towards long-term thinking and participatory democracy.

Conceptions of a Future Generations Act have often seen it as a mechanism to deliver the kind of civil and political rights embedded in the Human Rights Act – a constitutional protection should the government fail to meet targets around both global planetary health and global public health.[79] To this end, the legal duty should come alongside a range of government and accountability infrastructure – some of which can be adopted from Wales, a country that has pioneered this kind of legislation:

- An Office for Future Generations (OFG): To sit within government, with membership from Cabinet level ministers and accountable to the Prime Minister. The office should have an advisory role across local and national government, and there should be a duty on ministers to align policy to independently published OHG advice. The office should provide a counterbalance to the Treasury, which currently embeds an overly explicit focus on output growth, and policy short-termism.[80]
- Future Generations Assessments: Much as all policies make assessments on their economic and fiscal impact, a new future generations impact assessment should be introduced for all government spending decisions. This should pay reference to global planetary and health boundaries.
- A Future Generations Select Committee: The powerful role of select committees – otherwise, denigrated as stiff and dull meetings – has been seen during the pandemic. Their role in holding the health and social care secretaries to account, or in pulling Cameron over the coals after Greensill, has shown their role in ensuring accountability.[81] A new select committee should be set up to hold the government to account on its future generations obligations.
- A Permanent Health Sustainability Citizens Assembly: Future generations thinking means involving citizens from all generations. There is very little democratic participation on the UK's approach to health, whether local, national, or global. A standing citizens jury, drawn from representative samples of the country and

rotating annually, should work to both produce a steady stream of new ideas of global health sustainability, and to challenge the government on bad policy or inaction.

As with many policies on global health sustainability, these will need to be aligned with action on the highly related climate and nature emergencies. Done properly, they can help to ensure a healthy future for generations to come – and ensure the UK does its duty in extending that beyond its own, limited borders.

REGULATE FINANCE

Focusing on boundaries brings in scope finance. This is central to other agendas that focus on sustainability, such as climate and economic justice, and should also be a key consideration within public health sustainability.

In many cases, the relevant numbers are available from work focused on the climate emergency – but take on further urgency when also put in the context of global health sustainability. For instance, it remains the case, despite the rhetoric of financial companies from major banks and investment fund managers, that there is significant investment in fossil fuel companies. Research by the Rainforest Action Network has shown that the world's biggest banks have provided $3.8tn of financing for fossil fuel companies since the Paris Climate Accords (2016).[82] The evidence in this chapter shows these investments don't just constitute a risk to planetary health, but also to global public health.

The financial system provides scale and sustainability for sectors that drive other variables within my list of global health boundaries – beyond emissions. The role of the UK's high street banks in funding the arms trade is now well established. 2019 research from the organisation Facing Finance implicated some familiar high-street brands in supporting companies who have been linked to weapon exports in unstable/crisis affected countries in the Middle East and North Africa.[83] These included Deutsche Bank, Lloyds, Barclays and Santander – among others.[84]

If these facts are not new, what is novel is the opportunity to link these factors to infectious disease outbreaks. In Covid, we have proof that rich countries cannot 'safely' make money out of international conflict or climate emergency, without consequences to their own populations – the world is more interlinked than they've built into their cost-benefit analyses. Equally, we now have a case study of the consequences borne by an infectious disease outbreak – in terms of human and economic cost, nationally and internationally. The value in linking these factors to health is a strengthening of political capital, the weight of popularity and the cost-benefit analyses that can encourage political action.

There are a few structural factors that enable the financial system to underpin a breakdown in global health sustainability. Most obviously, there is little reason for banks to quantify and act on the health impacts of their investment. If a product they back causes chronic ill health, sustains foreign conflict and displacement, contributes to climate emergency through intensive emissions, or otherwise enters into activities that help concentrate wealth in Western countries and absolute poverty elsewhere, then neither the immediate cost, nor the long-term increased risk of infectious disease outbreak, need to be borne by banks or equity funds.

It is very difficult for this reason to bring these costs to the foreground. The size and power of banks makes them more difficult to regulate, as they have significant power in the face of states. Equally, it aggravates the size of mistakes. As the UK's initial Green New Deal Group argued in their work on defining the specifics of a Green New Deal, big banks make big mistakes.[85] And as the financial crisis showed, when financial institutions become 'too big to fail', they are more liable to take risks – like maintaining an approach to the sustainability of global public and planetary health that could plunge us into regular human, social and economic chaos.

After the pandemic, there is likely to be a pronounced focus on protecting the financial system from the risks posed by infectious diseases and health shocks. But what we really need is protection for global human health from the risks of the more unscrupulous tendencies of finance. That is, we need to bind the financial system to the boundaries of sustainable health, rather than further insulating its relentless search for growth from considerations of wider human flourishing.

In many cases, the specific policy instruments we need in global health policy can be adapted from those developed by the climate sector – particularly, from the excellent and innovative green finance movement. For instance, a combination of the Bank of England and the Treasury could look to use their lending schemes to leverage commercial banks to invest in projects that are sustainable from a global health perspective. Second, the UK's financial regulators could introduce measures that force financial institutions to account for pandemic risks. There will be no better time to do this, while private financial institutions count the cost of an unexpected health shock.

Elsewhere, tools in this book could be used to create health-specific financial targets. In 2021, the landmark report of the IPPR Environmental Justice Commission concluded that 'UK financial institutions should be legally required to set targets, including interim targets, to align their investments with net zero . . . '.[86] The PHN-ZERO makes a similar ambition possible, from a sustainability perspective, with financial firms challenged to ensure their portfolio does not make a net-negative impact on the global health boundaries.

MOBILISE PUBLIC RESEARCH AND DEVELOPMENT

The public sector had a starring role in generating a vaccine, a key achievement in the pandemic so far. While Prime Minister Boris Johnson said he thought the success was due to the 'greed of capitalism', the truer picture points to the contributions of public universities, publicly funded researchers, state investment, clinical researchers from the NHS and the National Health Service's ability to then distribute the vaccine across the country quickly.

Despite this, the public sector's contribution to global sustainability remains broadly untapped – particularly when it comes to generating new knowledge and innovation.

It's most undermined by a systematic lack of public investment. In 1986, the UK invested about 2 per cent of GDP in R&D per year – about the same as the average in other OECD nations. However, this year marked the first in a long-term decline. While OECD average investment in R&D activities has remained around 2 per cent per year, on average, UK investment has dropped to just over 1.5 per cent.[87] That means, over the course of 35 years, UK investment is £222 billion lower than if it had kept up with the average in other advanced economies.[88] This is puzzling, given the public popularity, economic boost and social value of science.

The political blocks to public investment in R&D since the 1980s are ideological. There remains an orthodoxy that the market can do things better (because of its supposedly greater efficiency in allocating resources). This suggests the role of the state is to get out of the way – in this case, it is argued that any unnecessary state involvement will 'crowd out' more efficient private sector activities.

Evidence has now discredited both ideas. First, it is very clear that the market needs help in allocating R&D investment to health priorities. For example, we might expect many diseases to receive a level of investment by the UK broadly in line with their burden on UK health.[89] But this is not the case. Cancer, renal, urogenital and skin conditions are receiving research investment in line with, or above, what their overall impact on health would suggest.[90] In other cases, conditions are missing out on significant research spend – chief amongst them the leading causes of both UK mortality (cardiovascular disease) and UK morbidity (neurological conditions and mental ill health). While an estimated £29 per person is invested in cancer research each year, only half as much goes into mental health research, despite it having a very similar overall burden on health. Just £9 per person goes into cardiovascular disease research. That represents a £650 million deficit for cardiovascular disease and a £350 million deficit for mental health conditions ever year.[91]

Second, research has shown that public investment does not simply replace or 'crowd out' private investment. In fact, the opposite is true. A 2016 study led by Jon Sussex showed that a 1 per cent increase in public sector investment in medical research was associated with a 0.81 per cent increase in private sector investment in research.[92] Where public investment goes, private sector investment follows. That only makes the value proposition for public-led R&D stronger – it means when it invests £1 in research, it can expect much more than £1 of research to take place.[93]

If we accept the case for a major programme of public sector investment and stewardship on health R&D, then a focus on pandemic prevention and sustainability is an obvious priority. Research by the Access to Medicines Foundation has demonstrated a severe lack of R&D on the priority pathogens that have the clearest epidemic potential. Having been struck by Covid-19, there is now lots of research on Covid-19 and coronaviruses, proxied by the 63 products in the R&D pipelines (i.e., future focused projects). Ebola and Zika, which have caused well-known outbreaks, have 5 and 4 items in their R&D pipeline. Chikungunya, Marburg and non-polio enteroviruses have 4, 1 and 1 projects in their pipeline respectively. And the ten other diseases on the list have no active R&D pipeline at all.

The reason is clear. The odds of any one of these diseases causing a shock event are very low – meaning there is little market today, and a very uncertain market for tomorrow. The impact they would have, however, and therefore the social need for research into them, is very high. This is a tailor-made area for the government to step in – and to use its historical underinvestment in R&D to rectify one of the biggest challenges we'll face in the future. This creates a distinct opportunity for the public sector to mobilise its existing resources, to help steer what kinds of research get done and to ensure the focus is on areas of greatest social priority. It would constitute a major and beneficial democratisation of health R&D.

6
The Public Health New Deal

The five frontiers of public health examined in the previous five chapters each proffer the potential for seismic shifts, both in improving the total stock of health in the country and in distributing that stock of health more justly.

Most ambitiously, the five frontiers in this book could be put together into a cohesive package through which to achieve radical advancement for our health. Taken together, this book constitutes a full blueprint for a healthy future: a public health new deal. We need arguments that go beyond the individual case for the policies discussed in the book so far. We need bespoke analysis on how such ideas fit together as a whole – not least, because the individual ideas together constitute an intervention an order of magnitude larger than anything discussed so far.

Three metrics strike me as particularly important. First, whether the blueprint is affordable. Second, whether a Public Health New Deal could be implemented without simply leaving us open to privatisation. And finally, whether we can balance the national nature of the public health new deal with the flexibility to adapt to the different material conditions of the local places and communities people actually live in.

* * *

There's no getting away from the fact that a Public Health New Deal is expensive. This is probably the most significant barrier to generating the political will and popular consensus needed to gain momentum and deliver real change.

Where ambitious and necessary ideas have come without a clear costing, they have sometimes been open to attack. At worst, reactive voices have seized the initiative by associating radical ideas with hyperbolic price tags. Often, it's little more than a cynical play to undermine public support. For example, the American Action Forum – a group suspicious of ambitious climate policy – undercut the US movement for a Green New Deal by attaching a costing of \$93 trillion to it in 2019.[1]

While their figure has not stood up to scrutiny, it has nonetheless proved damaging.

So, it's important to explore cost and affordability from the outset. This is simultaneously about policy substance and about communication. I'm aware the left is not in total agreement about how things should be funded – or, indeed, whether affordability is even meaningful. But even as we have these debates, we need to be realistic that a pragmatic price tag and justification for the investment is integral to the willingness of the public to support our suggestions for change. As such, the below constitutes a very safe estimate for costings, and whether they can be paid for – with the aim, at this early stage, of ensuring a concrete case for change.

COSTING THE NHS FRONTIER

In many cases, restoring the NHS from fragile safety net to comprehensive service would ensure a more efficient service in the long-term – either by improving the health of the country (and so boosting the economy), or by reducing the total cost of healthcare delivery.

Indeed, research shows large returns on investment are possible from expanding healthcare universality to the frontier of scientific possibility. Beyond the figures I've already cited in Chapter One, evidence indicates there are huge long-term returns on investment just waiting to be secured by extending universality in the NHS. For instance, estimates suggest that adopting the very best technology and AI could be worth £12.5 billion a year for the NHS – just because of the time it frees up for healthcare professionals.[2] Not only is this a significant sum of money, but healthcare professionals 'time to care' is the most valuable resource in health and care today.

None of this means that upfront investment wouldn't be necessary. The costs are often short-term, whilst the returns are mid–long term. Innovation – from new technology and new software, to digital tools – often has an upfront cost itself. But the more significant cost is often that of 'double running' services. The NHS cannot just end an old service before a new one gets up and running, as more often than not transformation relies on a patient period of running them in tandem.

One way to conceptualise the up-front investment we might need is to look at what comparable health systems with the best health outcomes deem necessary themselves. Despite our status as a G7 nation, and despite the popularity of NHS funding increases with the public, the UK spends significantly less on health than other countries (relative to GDP). Covid-19 emergency funding skews later statistics, but 2019 figures show that the UK spent around 10.25 per cent of GDP on health, compared to a G7 average of 11.5 per cent. Meeting the G7 average would imply increasing investment by an estimated £27.5 billion per year.[3]

This would provide the funds needed to deliver the four shifts outlined in Chapter One. The breakdown for this funding against the four components of extending universality could be:

1. **Bespoke Transformation Funding:** In 2020, IPPR research recommended a £10 billion transformation fund for the National Health Service could make a significant contribution to closing the gap in performance both within the country, and between the UK and comparable countries.[4]

2. **A Resilience Guarantee:** Many aspects of resilience will be achieved by other recommendations in the book – for example, public health advances will increase the population's health, likely putting us in better stead should health shocks (infectious or not) strike. Beds, community care and capital funding are three areas where funding is needed to deliver the 'resilience rules' discussed in Chapter 1. Combined, the evidence suggests that the current funding implications of a step-change in these areas would come to £3.4 billion per year.[5]

3. **Major Workforce Investment:** Pay justice for NHS workers could be achieved at a cost of £5.2 billion per year – sufficient for a 15 per cent pay rise. Outside of pay, a major uplift in mental health services for NHS workers could be achieved at an estimated cost of just £100 million.[6] In July 2020, a new scheme offered to cover childcare costs for GPs to boost recruitment. Expanding universal childcare across the NHS would cost an estimated £400 million.

4. **An Institutional Injustice Fund:** The remaining £8.4 billion per year should be allocated to radically driving forward access for people not currently well served by the NHS. Much of this funding should be focused on ensuring health services do not just sit back and wait for people to come in for care, but actively take care into the community. It should also look to significantly strengthen training and progression opportunities for people working in the NHS, who have

been systematically excluded from progression and leadership roles throughout the institution's history.

Table 6.1   Costing the NHS Frontier

Universalising the Best Expansion	Estimated Cost
Transformation fund	£10 billion per year
Resilience fund	£3.4 billion per year
Workforce fund	£5.7 billion per year
Inclusion health fund	£8.4 billion per year
Total	£27.5 billion per year

COSTING THE SOCIAL JUSTICE FRONTIER

The five prescriptions associated with a Universal Public Health Service are based on areas where strong evidence on cost and efficacy exist, often from the wider Universal Basic Services movement.

Inevitably, a first element of setting up the service will be a major expansion in headcount among existing public health teams. The Universal Public Health Service as a concept depends on the ability of public health professionals to build meaningful relationships with other local organisations and with communities themselves – within places, rather than as Whitehall body giving top-down diktats. The UK centralises more power than any other comparable country, and the policy prescriptions in this book should not be an excuse to further continue this centralisation.[7]

As such, the service would likely need a fleet of professionals operating in natural communities – not entirely different to a public health equivalent of the general practitioner, albeit designed around a social-prescription rather than a medical-prescription model. The proportion of existing public health budgets that go towards staffing costs is not systematically reported. Nonetheless we know that the NHS spends approximately 45 per cent of its total budget on staff pay (less during the pandemic years), and local councils a little more. It is reasonable to budget at a similar level here.

Costings for the five initial prescriptions for the Universal Public Health Service can then be estimated as follows:

1. A universal entitlement to a nutritious and sustainable diet has been costed at £1.5 billion per year.[8]
2. Social house building schemes have been costed at £1.2 billion in year 1 rising to £8.1 billion seven years later (and then lasting to year 30) by University College London.[9]
3. The cost of the education prescription can be estimated at £8 billion per year, based on extending existing investment in the pupil premium.[10]
4. Universalizing utilities, excluding digital access, has been costed at £5.1 billion per year elsewhere.[11] The additional inclusion of digital rebates has been costed at £300 million.[12]
5. Adapting existing costings for 'skill's wallet' schemes of £1.8 billion per year would give the Universal Public Health Service a budget equivalent to £10,000 per person/lifetime.
6. Given the unpredictable impact of Covid-19, an estimate for low pay and unemployment levels comes with significant uncertainty. Pre-Covid, giving public health professionals the ability to prescribe up to £500 per month to those receiving less than a minimum income standard would cost £11 billion per year (adjusted to account for elements of minimum income standards, like utilities, captured elsewhere).

These are likely to be long-run returns, both in terms of growth to the economy and reduced spending on other public services. For instance, NHS fiscal pressures might be reduced in the long-term, thanks to better population health and less avoidable illness. There are likely to be economic benefits from better health, on metrics like productivity, reduced absenteeism and reduced presenteeism. And there may also be decreases in the number of people relying on welfare payments as a consequence of poverty, too. As these benefits cannot be calculated with sufficient certainty to present here, and are unlikely to be realised in the short-term, the upfront investment is presented here without discount. As such, an estimated opening budget for the Universal Public Health Service is £39.2 billion.

In many cases, some of these costs will return almost immediately to the chancellor. For instance, a major expansion of jobs – in a period where unemployment is predicted to rise – would reduce reliance on unemployment benefits. Equally, public sector jobs are liable to income tax, national insurance and VAT on extra consumption, meaning much money returns to government. Estimates put the exact amount at between 50 and 80 per cent.[13] These discounts have not been applied here.

Table 6.2   Costing the Social Justice Frontier

Public Health Prescriptions	Estimated Cost
Universal nutrition prescription	£1.5 billion per year
Universal housing prescription	£1.2 billion in year 1, rising to 8.1 billion per year in year 8
Universal education prescription	£8 billion per year
Universal utilities prescription	£5.4 billion per year
Universal skills prescription	£1.8 billion per year
Universal work prescription	£11 billion per year
Expansion of public health teams	£13 billion per year
Total	c.£42 billion per year (initial)

COSTING THE ECONOMIC FRONTIER

The evidence shows that health taxes do not have a long-term impact on the business values of impacted companies and that a healthier workforce is likely to have its own economic value. Where taxes are enacted – including on public health harming practices like pollution, unhealthy food production, unscrupulous exploitation of mental health by social media, or discrimination of women and ethnic minorities when it comes to pay and progression – the revenues are likely to be substantial.

An exact measure of revenue potential is very hard to estimate (nor is it fixed). Two confounding factors are at play here. Firstly, as the case study of the soft drinks industry levy shows – in-line with other international health taxes and regulation – companies are often more likely to change their practices rather than pay taxes or pass it on to consumers. Most sugary drink producers did remove sugar from their products to avoid the levy – and, in fact, that was the whole idea. Second, as I point out in chapter three, exact targets and rates of tax would need to be established properly – most adequately by a unit of public health specialists sat either within the Treasury, the Cabinet Office or across Whitehall.

Nonetheless, the possibility of significant revenue – even with corporate behaviour change the primary aim – has a precedent. As of 2019, so-called 'green taxes' equalled 2.26 per cent of UK GDP – for a value of

approximately £60 billion per year.[14] Even this is not the limit of potential. Green taxes make up a much bigger percentage of GDP and share
of taxation in countries like Serbia, the Netherlands, Denmark and Italy.
Undeniably, public health taxes have similar potential: the government
commissioned National Food Strategy (2021) highlighted that nutrition
taxes alone could raise around £3 billion per year.[15]

Elsewhere, state monopolies could also generate significant revenue.
In 2017, estimates suggest Sweden's alcohol monopoly generated 29.4
billion SEK – or around £2.46 billion. That is revenue in a country with
a population about one sixth the size of the UKs, and one fifth the size of
England.[16] Meanwhile, the legal sale of marijuana is generating billions of
pounds in tax revenue alone, but even more in private profit – introducing a state monopoly would generate sizable funds. Applying the joint
potential of state sale and levies across a whole public health net zero
ambition suggests some potential to fund the whole package of investment outlined elsewhere in the book, or more.

Despite this, I do not put forward an arbitrary figure for what could be
raised, given the inevitable uncertainty that figure would rely on. We can
be confident that a good proportion – or, even, the whole of the proposal
recommended here – could be financed through these methods. But we
would not want our public health services to become overly reliant, or
worse, actively conditional, on revenue raised from negative corporate
health behaviours. The case for affordability is stronger if it can stand up
even without reference to the revenue raising potential of PHN-ZERO.

COSTING THE SOCIAL CARE FRONTIER

My proposals for social care begin from the existing consensus on the
left around a National Care Service, delivered on the same basis as the
National Health Service. The costs of Labour's 2019 social care commitments have been costed at £6 billion per year elsewhere.[17]

My evolution of these ideas combines the National Care Service with
ideas to help reform what care looks like – and what role it plays. The
recommendations which require investment are service double running
and a social care transformation fund. These could be linked to two
sources: first, calculations of the efficiencies possible by focusing care
on community-settings and independence (£2 billion per year),[18] and
the savings possible from the fact the new social care model will replace

NHS Continuing Healthcare funding (worth £3 billion per year).[19] This would imply setting the level of initial investment in transformation at approximately £5 billion per year.

This has a symmetry to President Joe Biden's recent stimulus package for community social care infrastructure, as part of his post-Covid $2 trillion stimulus package. His scheme invests $400 million over eight years to improve, expand and make resilient community and home care. The equivalent of this, once adjusted for the size of the UK economy and inflation, would be a major £40 billion investment in social infrastructure over an eight-year period.

On top of this, I estimate the cost of a carer dividend at £15 billion per year (as per Chapter Four).

Table 6.3   Costing the Social Care Frontier

Item	Estimated Annual Cost
Free personal care	£5 billion per year
Pay justice	£1 billion per year
Expansion of new care models	£5 billion per year
Unpaid care 'dividend'	£15 billion per year
Total	£26 billion per year

COSTING THE SUSTAINABILITY FRONTIER

The sustainability frontier makes one recommendation with notable expenditure implications. Namely, major public investment in R&D targeted at global public health challenges. Given the UK's cumulative underinvestment since the 1980s – £222 billion in total – a proportionate approach would be to rectify that over the same period, on top of existing plans. This process would make as much as £5 billion a year available for R&D on the structural drivers of global health and planetary health emergencies. This should be ring-fenced and must be over and above existing government spending ambitions.[20]

Brought together, this suggests the investment needed in setting up a Public Health New Deal would equal £100 billion. The hurdle we need to jump is whether this can be communicated as a reasonable or affordable amount of spending.

Table 6.4   Total Investment for a Public Health New Deal

Measure	*Estimated Extra Cost (Annually)*
NHS frontier	£27.5 billion per year
Social justice frontier	£42 billion in year 1, rising to 48.9 billion
Economic frontier	Revenue raising
Care frontier	£26 billion per year
Sustainability frontier	£5 billion per year
The Public Health New Deal	**c. £100–110 billion per year**

There are a few ways to communicate why this large amount of investment is reasonable.

First, we might point out that £100 billion doesn't even match the amount taken out of public finances during austerity. Research from 2019 shows that UK spending, as a percentage of GDP, was 8.1 per cent lower than the European average – which comes to approximately £230 billion.[21] The supposed upside of this policy was meant to be a stronger economy. However, other research, using figures produced by the Office for Budget Responsibility, has shown that the economy was £100bn smaller in 2018 than it would have been without public spending cuts.[22]

Second, we might point out how ambitious other countries have been on investment – compared to the UK – in the aftermath of the immediate Covid-19 shock. In the US, Joe Biden has led that agenda – with his $1.9 trillion stimulus package. The UK equivalent to a US stimulus would come to £190 billion (8.6 per cent of GDP).[23] Even then, the UK would not be the most ambitious country amongst those with similarly advanced economies. As early as December 2020, Japan announced a stimulus worth over 13 per cent of GDP. Converted to the UK, that would translate to a much bigger budget for economic stimulus still – somewhere between £250 and £300 billion. Such a sum could cover a Public Health New Deal, a UK Green New Deal and a significant amount of sustained support for people impacted[24] by the ongoing effects of the Covid-19 pandemic.[25]

Both these indicate the affordability of a Public Health New Deal. In one sense, it can be seen as a way to use public health to truly end austerity. In another, it can be a package through which the UK reacts proportionately to Covid, strengthens the economy, delivers growth, and prepares public services for an uncertain decade ahead. That is the economic and the health case both suggest the time is now ripe for a bold new deal style stimulus framed around, and justified through, public health.

ACHIEVABLE

In throwing our movement behind a radical new approach to health, we need to be confident that a shift away from a defensive, rear-guard defence on privatisation won't simply give a free hand to those who would destroy our NHS.

Having studied several private incursions into health and social care service in detail, there is a clear pattern.[26] The conditions for privatisation are most likely to emerge when the public sector faces false constraints which limit its ability to provide the best. That is, private health and care providers capitalise upon the failure to Universalise the Best.

In Winter and Spring, there was (rightly) an outcry from the left when Operose Health took over 37 more GP practices in London. Operose is a subsidiary of the US company Centene, and at the time the company already ran 21 GP practices in England. This new incursion took its total to 58. This means, at the time of writing, this large, for-profit company controlled the care of 500,000 patients. It is the biggest single primary care provider in the country.

The unified position on the left was the correct one: Operose must be stopped and immediately barred from delivering healthcare services for profit. Just as I have shown in social care, large operators are poorly suited to provide effective, efficient, and ethical health and care services.

But once a private provider has managed to infiltrate the NHS, it is far harder to get rid of them. The fact that we only realised the Operose threat *after* they had taken a significant market share makes our campaigns far more difficult. And while we could put this down to the sneakiness of American corporate interests, or on backdoor dealing within government, this might lack some necessary self-reflection. The signs of trouble – and the conditions that lead to privatisation – were visible long before most on the left had ever heard of Operose.

When privatisation happens, we on the left tend to ask the same three questions:

1. How did a private company manage to infiltrate the NHS?
2. What are the downsides of this privatisation?
3. How can we can reverse it?

We are less good at working out the conditions that lead to privatisation, and the right strategies to prevent it from ever happening – rather than just reacting to it.

Therefore the most important question is the one asked the least often: what conditions allowed Operose Health to successfully buy so many GP practices? While the answer doesn't help us get them out of our healthcare system now, it does teach us vital lessons about how their incursion was allowed to occur. And that is vital in preventing it from happening again.

To answer the question adequately we need to begin with a little primary care history. GPs have always worked on a slightly different basis to the rest of the NHS. Whereas other medical professionals are usually employed on an NHS contract, GPs are often self-employed. Traditionally, practices are run by GP partnerships. They are run as a business: employing their own staff, managing their premises and delivering services for the NHS on an independent contractor basis.

In 1948, the model was seen to have advantages worth keeping. Specifically, it was felt that leaving general practitioners to work as partners in small practices would have two benefits: i) innovation – partners with a financial stake would have skin in the game, and an incentive to adopt best practices; ii) localism – in a very centralised system, it was hoped that GPs would understand their patients and tailor the NHS to meet their needs.

It was also useful from a political perspective. Bevan faced opposition to his NHS Bill from the medical unions and the opposition parties. Maintaining the GP status quo helped ensure the legislation passed.

Seventy years later, our system of small, business-owning GPs has reached breaking point. Even before Covid-19, general practice was facing a crisis of workload. Surveys by the British Medical Association regularly showed the immense pressure facing GPs in particular – with 63 per cent of clinicians indicating the workload in their practices as 'unmanageable' in January 2020.[27] By 2021, Pulse found GPs were working eleven-hour days on average.[28]

This is bad for patients. Such sharp rises in workload, predictably, have consequences for access. In 2020, my research showed that 36 per cent of people in England were waiting more than a week for a GP appointment. And 3 per cent of people were not able to book an appointment at all, the last time they needed one. That won't immediately hit anyone as a massive number, but it's nonetheless the equivalent of 1.7 million people in England going without access to their GP.[29] Given General Practice provides the gateway to the rest of the NHS, that means severely limited access to the whole gamut of healthcare.

Working in a broken system is severely harming GP numbers. Despite government efforts to recruit more people into general practice – including a golden handshake policy, where new GPs were rewarded with an immediate £10,000 – the number of GPs in England per 100,000 people has reached its lowest level since 2003. Compared to 2003, the population has much more chronic, complicated health needs – meaning the same numbers per person translates to significantly less GP capacity.

The simple arithmetic is this: people are retiring from general practitioner roles more quickly than people are entering the profession. Not enough prospective doctors want to become GPs. It has become a profession associated with poor reward, linear careers, overwork and stress. It perfectly epitomises the worst of the worrying workforce trends I worked through in Chapter One.

Those left in the profession are taking proactive steps to manage their own workload and burnout. In 2015, the average GP worked the equivalent of 0.84 FTE (full-time equivalent). In 2019, that had dropped to 0.76 FTE.[30] That drop is the equivalent of losing a whole 3,000 GPs – in just four years. Faced with a major increase in work, GPs are choosing to work part-time to manage their work/life balance. That is entirely understandable.

The decline in GP numbers comes with a hidden sting in the tail. It means that there are less and less people willing to take over a GP practice, when one of the existing 'partners' comes to sell. In the worst cases, this leads to a 'last person standing' problem – whereby a skeleton crew of GP partners who want to stop working simply cannot, because they are financially bound to their practice, and unable to pass it on. They are locked in.

This brings us back to Operose. Having done extensive research on primary care, I've had the chance to talk candidly to many people working in senior Operose roles. I often hear the same remarks. They tell me that General Practitioners are coming to them, sometimes in quite desperate and unhappy circumstances, and pleading with them to take over the practice. They might be doing it so they can retire. They might be doing it because the workload is simply too much – and they want to pass on the practice management to someone else, while continuing to focus on clinical duties. Without Operose, their only way out may very well be financial ruin.

So, a big corporate entity has become the only route of escape for doctors desperate to get out of the sector with their health and finances intact. A sub-optimal model of organising general practice, a workforce crisis and limited patient access to services are the determinants of privatisation. That is, privatisation slips into the gaps where state provision and best practice separate – in the growing areas where Universalise the Best is not secure.

The more proactive strategy for preventing privatisation would have been a simple expansion of Bevan's fundamentals: nationalisation of GPs. In early 2020, just months before the Operose takeover, I proposed this very policy – delivered through a right to NHS (i.e., public sector) employment for all current general practitioners and compulsory NHS employment for all new general practitioners. This would have immediately ensured several improvements:

- Pay: GPs earn less in this country than elsewhere. Average pay should be aligned to international averages.
- Flexibility: GPs currently have poor access to flexible working, with anecdotal evidence indicating many struggles not only to take lunch breaks, but toilet breaks. Flexible working should be key to a new role, with aspirations to use any boost in recruitment to cut the GP working week.
- Variation: GPs today do not want to just rush patient to patient. They want to do research, leadership, strategy and a host of other valuable activities. All GPs should have the right to combine their role with another activity, as part of a portfolio career.

These were proposals developed after extensive consultation with GPs, looking to understand their aspirations, needs and experiences of the system today. It was oriented towards benefitting workers and, in turn, alleviating the difficulties with access emerging from dire recruitment and retention in general practice. That is, it was developed from the realisation that if the state didn't act, it was only a matter of time before the private sector did.

A frontier approach to health, based on universalising the best, would allow us to implement the policies necessary to avoid privatisation. A defensive, rear-guard action forces us to wait until it happens, and only then react.

In fact, our movement can sometimes be its own worst enemy.[31] We could have prevented privatisation by nationalising GPs. This would be a major change to the status quo. And yet, despite the fact it is a move so in-line with the evidence and with Bevan's principles, the idea of changing the model of general practice is fiercely opposed by the key institutions of the health labour movement: royal colleges and trade unions. Both are staunch defenders of the status quo in general practice, as broken as it is.[32] Both put out media statements dismissing the nation-alisation policy – six months later, Centene was the biggest GP operator in the country.

We need our own compelling vision for the future. Otherwise, we will simply find ourselves defending the way things are, even as they break. And it is those breaks through which private companies can slip in. The Public Health New Deal is about avoiding this, at scale, across public health as a whole.

PLACE

Clement Attlee's Labour government did not all agree on what format the National Health Service should take. One side of the debate was taken up by Nye Bevan, who was convinced of the merits of a national system – famously declaring that the sound of a dropped bedpan in Tredegar should reverberate around Whitehall. The case for a much more locally led health service was championed by the Leader of the House of Commons, Lord President of the Council and future Deputy Leader of the Opposition: Herbert Morrison.

A former leader of London County Council, Morrison set out on a quest to convince colleagues that the health service should be run from local councils. His case relied on a few arguments. First, he said that taking cherished and long-standing functions like health away from local authorities would severely diminish their power. Second, he argued that it would install a one-size-fits-all system, making it much harder to meet the different health needs of different places.

Bevan, as we know, won out. He convinced colleagues that a centrally funded National Health Service should equally be controlled by central government. And he won the argument that a *national* service would be more equal and more efficient than a more locally led NHS, which would allow a postcode lottery to emerge.

In thinking about how the Public Health New Deal is implemented, it is important to consider the level at which it will be led. I believe there is a balance to be struck here. In principle, the Public Health New Deal is a national proposition. Like the NHS, it is driven by the idea that a central proposition applicable to the whole country is key to both the popularity of the policy, and its ability to deliver justice. Throughout, the principles driving a new blueprint are that the right to good health, for free, can be expanded within and beyond the NHS.

However, we cannot ignore that our health is defined by the material conditions of the places in which we live. We can see this at different levels of geographical analysis. From a regional perspective, the data shows us that health and care needs cluster in the North and the Midlands. Take, for example, the rate at which people die of ill health before they reach their seventy-fifth birthday – a concept used to indicate 'premature' mortality in health statistics (that is, mortality that should be prioritised as avoidable with the best preventative and medical practices).

Table 6.5 Under 75 Mortality Rate per 100,000 Population, England, By Region[33]

	All Causes	CVD	Cancer	Respiratory Disease	Stroke	Liver Disease
North East	394.74	82.80	152.60	44.20	16.31	25.5
North West	388.39	86.60	145.60	46.30	15.20	25.7
Yorkshire and the Humber	363.18	82.00	141.20	41.20	14.29	19
East Midlands	334.42	73.50	133.40	34.90	12.62	17.5
West Midlands	354.41	78.40	138.30	36.30	13.28	21.3
East	302.12	63.40	126.00	29.80	11.56	15
London	303.32	70.50	120.10	30.30	13.13	16
South East	292.31	59.00	123.60	28.70	10.72	15.7
South West	301.46	61.90	125.60	28.10	11.19	15.9
England	330.49	71.7	132.3	34.7	12.83	18.5

The shading in Table 6.5 show where a region has a mortality rate before age 75 per 100,000 people above the England average. If each shaded box counted as one point, the North and Midlands would have a score of 28 out 30 – representing the fact that the East Midlands has *just* lower than average mortality from stroke and liver disease. By contrast, the East and South of the country would score just one point out of a possible 24 – with London having above average premature mortality from stroke.

Underneath this regional analysis is a clustering of ill health in smaller places. At local authority level, of the ten places with the highest rates of mortality considered preventable from cardiovascular, respiratory disease, liver disease, stroke and cancer, six areas are in the top ten for all five conditions and a further two for four conditions.[34] These places are overwhelmingly outside the more affluent South East of the country, and places where socio-economic deprivation is highest. It strongly suggests a one-size-fits-all approach to health won't work, if only because it does not address the systemic injustices of the country as we find it today.

The interaction between place and health was made very clear by Covid. Almost exactly two years after Boris Johnson introduced 'levelling up' as a key rhetorical theme of his leadership – during the Conservative leadership election in 2019 – Professor Sir Michael Marmot released new analysis exploring the disproportionate impact Covid-19 had had across the country in 2020. His analysis showed that mortality had been 25 per cent higher in Greater Manchester than in England as a whole. As a result, life expectancy had fallen faster in the North West that year than in the rest of England. And a close relationship between deprivation and Covid mortality meant that a fall in life expectancy had been focused on both the poorest parts of England and the poorest parts of the North West region.

This is all to say that we need to have a much stronger conception of the role of place – in designing, delivering and tailoring this major new public health plan – than there was when the NHS was formed.

The key to a workable place-based approach to the Public Health New Deal is two-fold. First, we need a plan that genuinely redistributes power over health – to people and local leaders, to co-create services in places together. Second, we need a firm appreciation of the material conditions implicit in place and a plan for ensuring that our investment in health provides an anchor and a source of community development for the places that need it most. That is to say, the level of investment implicit in a Public Health New Deal can be a public health intervention itself – above and beyond the specific services it funds – because of its capacity to catalyse regeneration in the parts of the country worst hit by Thatcherism, deindustrialisation and austerity.

We do not need to begin from scratch. There are a range of models that can provide a basis for implementing the Public Health New Deal – nationally – in a way that is cognisant of the different material conditions of place.

For example, the last decade saw Wigan embark on a major process of change, towards a model of 'asset-based working at scale'.[35] The subsequently named 'Wigan Deal' was based on a new relationship between public services and local people. First the council and its partners engaged in intensive, local interviews over a week-long period. They mapped out its services, its voluntary sector, its citizens' capabilities and its leadership. It developed a system where public sector workers had permission to innovate, where a dedicated community investment fund could fund community development and where council service commissioning was more collaborative.[36] It has been remarkably successful, with health and social care improved, financial sustainability maintained despite the severity of austerity's cuts and improved wellbeing outcomes for citizens.[37]

Outside of health, other place-based schemes provide a basis for using the investment implicit in a Public Health New Deal to deliver community regeneration. In Preston, the now famous 'Preston Model' was developed under the leadership of councillor Matthew Brown, who heads the council. The Preston model is an initiative formed on building community wealth through a different type of economics of place. Having found that 56 per cent of spend from 'anchor institutions' – vital public services, with big procurement, delivery and employment footprints – had left the region, Preston acted. It began a large-scale influencing project, pushing their public services to procure from local and socially responsible suppliers. Procurement processes and documents were overhauled, to ensure these suppliers could win contracts.

It is a model of regeneration that keeps money in the local economy, and ensures it reaches local people. City council staff receive at least a living wage and play a role in advocating for its adoption across employers. The amount of procurement spend staying in Preston has more than doubled since 2012/13. The co-operative sector has grown. Major housing and commercial real estate developments are required to provide skills and employment plans for local people.[38]

Preston is the most famous example of a social-value approach to regeneration and a local-retention approach to spending. But it is not the only such example. Salford's mayor Paul Dennett has pioneered a model of 'sensible socialism' that is also reaping dividends. This has included a council-owned development company to drive social housing; a similar focus on anchor institutions and social value standards to Preston; and a regime of borrowing at low interest rates to invest in the local economy, infrastructure and carbon footprint.[39]

These kinds of schemes suggest several lessons in how place can feature in the implementation and value-maximisation of a major investment in public health:

- Investment should be kept within places, particularly those where socio-economic deprivation is the highest
- Regulation associated with the Public Health Net Zero and services associated with the Universal Public Health Service should be based on established principles of community wealth building
- New public health, care and health services should be done *with* people, through sustained engagement – rather than done *to* them, in a paternalistic fashion
- In implementing the deal, there should be a focus on local employment, supporting socially valuable enterprises, developing and involving community assets and building partnerships – things that are good for public health, above and beyond what new services are launched
- The £100 billion should not be controlled exclusively by Whitehall, but used to empower local leaders as much as possible – in line with the well-established principles of devolution in health and care

While the entitlement to good health is national, and while the Public Health New Deal is a national solution to a problem we all face, the value of the deal will only be realised in full if it works with places, in the context of the material conditions of places, and uses its investment to create thriving communities of people above and beyond the specific services it implements.

A HEALTHY FUTURE IS POSSIBLE

When I talk to people about the future of health, there is often a sense of pessimism. They wonder how much longer general taxation can support the NHS in the face of growing health need. They wonder how we'll catch-up with the health outcomes of our international peers. They fret about the trajectory of a social care support system mired by crisis. They predict widening inequality, a second bout of austerity and continued reversals in healthy life expectancy and longevity.

Public perceptions research shows that this pessimism isn't unique to my friends and colleagues. As much as the country love the NHS, they are fearful about the future. 81 per cent of the public think our health system is overstretched. In other countries, the average number who think their own national health system is stretched is just 55 per cent.[40] Polling has also shown that the public think health services are getting worse, and a similar amount think the general standard of care will get worse in the near future.[41] There is little optimism about health and care.

But if I've argued for anything over the last few hundred pages, it is that a healthy future is possible. Good health remains one of the greatest, untapped resources for a just society and a just economy – locally and nationally. It is possible to come up with a positive vision for how we can unleash that potential following the greatest health shock the country has experienced in its modern history.

It was from the destruction of war that the NHS was born. The charge for such a radical policy was led by popular writers and radicals, George Orwell among them. From the ashes of Covid-19, we need the same level of radical change. Once again, we face the stark realities of sub-optimal health and rife health injustice.

This decade sees us at a crossroad. Two futures are possible. One will see the status quo sustained. The NHS will be strained, inequalities will widen, life expectancy will fall back and elderly people will continue to suffer in care homes. The other offers a radical advancement of public health, a reinvention of Bevan's democratic socialism over five frontiers. With it will come a fairer economy, social justice and greater sustainability.

It's no longer enough to maintain the status quo. In this desperately uncertain moment, we must be bold in reaching out and grasping it. Only then is a healthier, fairer future possible.

Epilogue
Labour's Medicine

I have not spoken much about Labour Party strategy in this book. I have not wanted to suggest the Parliamentary Labour Party are the only route to change, nor that they are synonymous with the left and its movements. Nonetheless, as the UK's biggest progressive political party there is no doubt that they're important. It is worth considering how the ideas outlined in this book fit with their agenda and electoral prospects.

Health has long been a foundation of the Labour Party's electoral strategy. Under some very different leaders – from a full array of the coalition that makes up the 'Parliamentary Labour Party' – it has campaigned on its ability to steward the nation's health service and improve the nation's health. In the same way the Conservatives have dined on their reputation in governing 'the economy', Labour have presented themselves as 'the party of the NHS'.

Historically, this approach has served the Labour Party well. Winning on health has allowed it to capitalise on an issue at the very heart of what people care about, and that genuinely impacts on how they have cast their vote.

The market research company Ipsos Mori have created monthly 'issues indexes' now for decades. My analysis of their polling shows that, when the polls were first carried out, the NHS was considered something of a fringe issue. In the first month, it was selected as most important by just 3 per cent of the public. The next month, just 2. The importance of the NHS rose steadily through the next decade. By 1988, it was the most important issue for a massive 64 per cent of voters. In the three decades since, health has been the most consistent priority issue for the public.

Health may well be *the* defining issue in deciding modern elections.

In recent times, Labour have tended to do well at the ballot box when they've been successful at putting the NHS at the top of the agenda. In his own analysis of Ipsos polling data, health and care commentator Richard Sloggett suggests two things have predicted Labour election victories recently. First, the NHS being listed as important by more than 40 per cent of voters. Second, the NHS rising in importance during the election campaign period.[1]

In 2010, the NHS fell in importance for voters during the election campaign (- 2 per cent) and was listed as important by only a quarter of voters. Throughout Gordon Brown's premiership, voter prioritisation of healthcare hit lows not seen since the early 1980s. Labour recorded a historic loss. In 1997 and 2017, where Labour broke 40 per cent of the national vote, the NHS recorded massive increases in salience during the election campaign window: 14 and 13 per cent respectively.

The implication is that the Labour Party have not been able to win without health and, unless something changes quite dramatically, are significantly less likely to win without health in the future. And so, it should worry their strategists deeply that there have been signs that the Labour Party are beginning to lose their advantage on health. Despite an exception in 2017 – where Labour's narrative was far more nuanced than in 2019 – the party's story isn't resonating quite as well or widely as it used to (*Table E.1*).

Table E.1   Labour Lead on Healthcare Ahead of Election[2]

Year	Labour lead on healthcare among all voters	% Mentioning healthcare as important	Increase (%) from month before	Labour vote share
2019 (December)	+12	55	+ 1	32.2
2017 (June)	+14	61	+ 13	40.0
2015 (May)	+13	44	+ 3	30.4
2010 (May)	+9	22	+ 2	29.0
2005 (May)	+12	36	+ 8	35.2
2001 (June)	+28	58	+ 17	40.7
1997 (May)	+32	63	+ 24	43.2
1992[3] (April)	+23	41	+ 8	34.4

These figures suggest performance on health in the lead up to elections is a strong predictor of election outcome. The trend seems to be that the manner in which health, as an agenda, supports a Labour election victory is a product of three things: a large Labour lead; lots of public salience; and a decent rise in salience in the general election campaigning period (when people who normally don't obsess about politics are tuning in more intensely).

We might group the election results in Table E.1 into three broad groups.

- Group One (Over 40% vote share): Labour manage to mobilise the health and care as a key issue through the campaign, people list health and care as a key issue, and Labour are rewarded with a big lead on the issue. (1997, 2001, 2017)
- Group Two (30-40% vote share): Healthcare is seen as important and Labour obtain a moderate lead, but do not manage to increase salience of the agenda in the election campaign window (2015, 2005, 1992)
- Group Three (below 30% vote share): Labour don't manage to mobilise health as a key issue, people don't list health as a key issue, and Labour don't have a big lead on the issue (2010)

The low-tens and high single-digit figure leads on healthcare that Labour saw in the 2010s are reminiscent of the 1980s – Thatcher's decade of dominance, and a decade of misery for the Labour Party. Then, Thatcher was very good at constraining Labour's lead on health – and in reducing their lead on health during general election campaigns. She managed to cut it by 18 points from previous peaks, in the period directly preceding the 1983 and 1987 elections.

The political right's strategists evidently sense that Labour's strength on health is waning. There is a real belief at Conservative Party HQ and in Number 10 that they can win on health consistently – and in doing so negate one of their historic problem areas. They have demanded that Conservative MPs and officials get in line with the idea of a publicly funded health service, even if they don't particularly like it. Where the NHS was once considered a toxic topic for Conservatives, it has now become one of their key lines. Prime Minister Boris Johnson has shown a particular predilection for putting health at the heart of his campaigning – including during the referendum on Britain's membership of the EU (£350 million/week) and in the 2019 general election (where the NHS was positioned as *the* thing we could turn to once the country 'got Brexit done').

In tandem, the right has begun to more strongly challenge the narrative that they are a risk to the NHS, namely by highlighting how they've been in charge for most of its existence (now, 43 of its 73 years).[4] There have even been incursions to Labour's 'home turf'. One of the 2019 TV leader debates saw Boris Johnson successfully attack Jeremy Corbyn on the role of Private Finance in the NHS despite Jeremy Corbyn being a staunch critique of PFI and Johnson having been a minister in governments that had actively used the scheme.

The recent years of Conservative Party dominance have been defined by remarkable ideological agility. They have positioned themselves as the party of common sense, of generational equality and the party of the working class. Now they are positioning themselves, with some success, as the party of the NHS and health more widely. And just as presenting Labour as a party of good economic governance helped Blair win elections, so could managing to present themselves as a party of good health governance help the right create further electoral success.

The canary in the coalmine for the success of their approach is the willingness of NHS workers to vote Conservative. According to polling undertaken by Nursing Notes, 42 per cent of healthcare workers voted for the Conservative Party during the local elections in 2021.[5] That figure is despite the run up to the election being dominated by government failures on Covid-19, and a scandal around a proposed post-Covid pay rise for NHS workers of just 1 per cent.

The challenging reality is that the Labour Party need a far more compelling vision and story when it comes to health, and to create new political divides and a vision unique to leftist politics. They need to speak far more about why right-wing politics undermines resilience in the NHS. They need to speak of how the crisis in care stems from political ideology, not just incompetence. Most of all, they need to speak about how the conditions of social injustice, and the exploitations of capital and structure of our economy, make us all sick – and disproportionately kill the poorest and least powerful in our society.

In short, they need to do far better at meeting people where they are and engaging with the lived reality of health. This is how they can reinvigorate the health agenda, and present good health as something only Labour can provide – at a time when both parties are willing to pump large sounding funding numbers into healthcare.

The Labour Party cannot survive if they lose health. It's time for them to adopt a radical new blueprint for the future of public health.

Notes

All articles last accessed 8 September 2021.

PREFACE

1. Clare Wenham, 'What is the future of UK leadership in global health security post Covid-19?', *Progressive Review*, 27/2 (2020), onlinelibrary. wiley.com/doi/full/10.1111/newe.12201.
2. Jacqueline Rose, 'Pointing the finger', *London Review of Books*, 7 May 2020, www.lrb.co.uk/the-paper/v42/n09/jacqueline-rose/pointing-the-finger.
3. See, for example Grace Blakeley, 'Capitalism's covid recovery will deepen social inequality', *Tribune*, 13 April 2021, www.tribunemag.co.uk/2021/04/ capitalisms-covid-recovery-will-deepen-social-inequality.

INTRODUCTION

1. The point at which he adopted his more famous penname, George Orwell.
2. A hospital that still exists today, albeit with a much-enhanced reputation.
3. George Orwell, 'How the Poor Die', (1946). Available at: www. orwellfoundation.com/the-orwell-foundation/orwell/essays-and-other-works/how-the-poor-die/.
4. Over 39.4 degrees Celsius, well above the 38 degree threshold for a fever.
5. Orwell, 'How the Poor Die'.
6. Ibid.
7. Notably, 'How the Poor Die' was first published in the same year Bevan brought his NHS bill before parliament (1946).
8. *The Sunday Express*, 'We're all in this together and can beat coronavirus', editorial, 15 March 2020, www.express.co.uk/comment/expresscomment/ 1255323/coronavirus-outbreak-UK-Government-measures-latest-death-toll.
9. John Harris, 'Coronavirus means we really are, finally, all in this together', *Guardian*, 29 March 2020, www.theguardian.com/commentisfree/2020/ mar/29/coronavirus-means-we-really-are-finally-all-in-this-together.
10. *Evening Standard*, 'A rainbow of hope as London stands together', editorial, 25 March 2020, www.standard.co.uk/comment/comment/evening-standard-comment-a-rainbow-of-hope-as-london-stands-together-a4397296.html.
11. See Toyin Owoseje, 'Coronavirus is "the great equalizer," Madonna tells fans from her bathtub', *CNN*, 23 March 2020, www.edition.cnn.com/2020/03/23/ entertainment/madonna-coronavirus-video-intl-scli/index.html.

12. Public Health England, *Disparities in the risk and outcomes of COVID-19*, August 2020, https://assets.publishing.service.gov.uk/government/uploads/system/uploads/attachment_data/file/908434/Disparities_in_the_risk_and_outcomes_of_COVID_August_2020_update.pdf.

13. Ibid. p. 39.

14. Author's analysis of Office for National Statistics, *Coronavirus (COVID-19) related deaths by occupation, England and Wales*, dataset, 2021, www.ons.gov.uk/peoplepopulationandcommunity/healthandsocialcare/causesofdeath/datasets/coronaviruscovid19relateddeathsbyoccupationenglandandwales. Figures given for men, with data for deaths among women involving Covid-19 by occupation far more limited. The data that does exist coheres to this trend.

15. Ibid.

16. Hannah E. Davis, Gina S. Assaf, Lisa McCorkell et al., 'Characterising long COVID in an international cohort: 7 months of symptoms and their impact', *EClinicalMedicine*, 38/101019 (August 1, 2021), https://doi.org/10.1016/j.eclinm.2021.101019.

17. Office for National Statistics, *Prevalence of ongoing symptoms following coronavirus (COVID-19) infection in the UK: 1 July 2021*, 2021, www.ons.gov.uk/peoplepopulationandcommunity/healthandsocialcare/conditionsanddiseases/bulletins/prevalenceofongoingsymptomsfollowingcoronaviruscovid19infectionintheuk/1july2021.

18. Ibid.

19. See Mick Tucker and Paul Kenyon, 'Long Covid pay decision for key workers could take a year', *BBC*, 18 May 2021, www.bbc.co.uk/news/uk-57146120.

20. Healthy life expectancy is an official measure of life lived in 'reasonable' health. It takes into account quality of life as well as longevity.

21. Office for National Statistics, *Health state life expectancies by national deprivation deciles, England and Wales: 2017 to 2019*, data release, 22 March 2021, www.ons.gov.uk/peoplepopulationandcommunity/healthandsocialcare/healthinequalities/bulletins/healthstatelifeexpectanciesbyindexofmultipledeprivationimd/2017to2019.

22. Theresa A. Hestert et al., 'Disparities in cancer incidence and mortality by area-level socioeconomic status: a multilevel analysis', *Journal of Epidemiology and Community Health*, 69/2, (2015): 168–176. Doi: 10.1136/jech-2014-204417.

23. Author's calculations. As this book enters production in July 2021, where most adults have been vaccinated, the figure is 1 in every 33 Covid deaths globally. But this has only been enabled by a vaccination inequality that has allowed many rich countries to double-jab their least vulnerable before less wealthy countries have really even begun their own programmes. Data analysis uses official population estimates and John Hopkin's Covid-19 tracker: https://coronavirus.jhu.edu/data/cumulative-cases. (Accessed 28 February 2021 and 12 July 2021).

24. Harry Quilter-Pinner, 'The hidden cost of Covid-19 on the NHS – and how to "build back better"', Institute for Public Policy Research, 16 August 2020, www.ippr.org/blog/the-hidden-cost-of-covid-19-on-the-nhs.

25. Parth Patel, Chris Thomas and Harry Quilter-Pinner, *Without skipping a beat*, Institute for Public Policy Research, 2021, www.ippr.org/research/publications/without-skipping-a-beat.

26. Parth Patel, Chris Thomas and Harry Quilter-Pinner, *The state of health and care: The NHS long term plan after Covid-19*, Institute for Public Policy Research, 2021, www.ippr.org/research/publications/state-of-health-and-care

27. Andrew Hood, Thomas Jemmmett and Victor Yu, 'Mental health surge model', *The Strategy Unit*, November 2020, www.strategyunitwm.nhs.uk/mental-health-surge-model

28. UCL, 'Majority feel they comply with Covid-19 Rules better than others', 4 December 2020, www.ucl.ac.uk/news/2020/dec/majority-feel-they-comply-covid-19-rules-better-others; University College London, 'Lockdown compliance improving but low take up of Covid tests "worrying"', 13 January 2021, www.ucl.ac.uk/news/2021/jan/lockdown-compliance-improving-low-take-covid-tests-worrying.

29. Marina Sitrin (ed.), *Pandemic solidarity: Mutual aid during the Covid-19 crisis*, Pluto Press, 2020.

30. Friedrich Engels and Karl Marx, *The communist manifesto*, translated by Samuel Moore, Penguin Books, 2002 [1848], p. 225.

31. Milton Friedman, *Capitalism and freedom*, University of Chicago Press, p. xiv.

32. Centre for Systems Science, *Covid-19 dashboard*, www.arcgis.com/apps/opsdashboard/index.html#/bda7594740fd40299423467b48e9ecf6.

33. Office for National Statistics, 'Coronavirus and the impact on output in the UK Economy: December 2020', 12 February 2021, www.ons.gov.uk/economy/grossdomesticproductgdp/articles/coronavirusandtheimpactonoutputintheukeconomy/december2020#:~:text=6.,The%20UK%20economy%20during%20the%20coronavirus%20(COVID%2D19)%20pandemic,to%20the%20measurement%20of%20GDP.

34. Gyongyosi Gyozo and EmilVerner, 'Financial crisis, creditor-debtor conflict and political extremism', *Beltrage zur Jahrestagung des Vereains fur Socialpolitik, Digitale Wirtschaft – Session: International Financial Markets*, (April 2021), http://dx.doi.org/10.2139/ssrn.3289741.

35. More recently, the party have changed their name to National Rally.

36. Manuel Funke, Moritz Schularick and Christoph Trebesch, 'Going to extremes: Politics after financial crises, 1870 – 2014', *European Economic Review*, 88/1 (2016): 227–260.

37. Kristian Blickle, 'Pandemics change cities: Municipal spending and voter extremism in Germany, 1918-1933', *Federal Reserve Bank of New York Staff Reports*, 921 (May 2020), www.newyorkfed.org/medialibrary/media/research/staff_reports/sr921.pdf

38. Mark A. Senn, 'English life and law in the time of the Black Death', *Real Property, Probate and Trust Journal*, 38/3 (2003): 507–588; Elizabeth Bruenig, 'If Anti-Vaxxers want a revolution, they just might get one', *New*

Republic, 4 February 2015, www.newrepublic.com/article/120960/ disease-epidemics-have-long-history-causing-political-upheaval.

39. R. J. Evans, 'Epidemics and revolutions: Cholera in nineteenth-century Europe', *Past & Present*, 120 (August 2020): 123–146.

40. Reginald E. Zelnik, *Labor and society in Tsarist Russia*, Stanford University Press, 1971.

41. Documented in leaked emails from June.

42. Neena Modi, 'Health systems should be publicly funded and publicly provided', *British Medical Journal*, 10/362 (2018), https://doi.org/10.1136/bmj.k3580.

43. Florien M. Kruse et al., 'Do private hospitals outperform public hospitals regarding efficiency, accessibility and quality of care in the European Union? A literature Review', *The International Journal of Health Planning and Management*, 33/2 (2018): 434–453, onlinelibrary.wiley.com/doi/full/10.1002/hpm.2502.

44. Sonia Adesara and Chris Thomas, 'Environmental collapse means more crises are coming – how can the NHS resist?', *IPPR Progressive Review*, 27/3 (2020), onlinelibrary.wiley.com/doi/abs/10.1111/newe.12208; Neena Modi, 'Health systems should be publicly funded and publicly provided'.

45. Ben Clover and Katherine Hignett, 'NHS braces for £10bn spend on outsourcing work to private hospitals', *The Health Service Journal*, 2020, www.hsj.co.uk/finance-and-efficiency/nhs-braces-for-10bn-spend-on-outsourcing-work-to-private-hospitals/7028255.article.

46. Mark Dayan and Helen Buckingham, 'Will the new Health and Care Bill privatise the NHS?', *Nuffield Trust*, 15 July 2021, www.nuffieldtrust.org.uk/news-item/will-the-new-health-and-care-bill-privatise-the-nhs.

47. It probably was in the 1980s, when there were very lively discussions among the Thatcher government about making denationalisation of the NHS official government policy.

48. House of Commons, *National Health Service Bill: Order for second reading*, Hansard, 30 April 1946, api.parliament.uk/historic-hansard/commons/1946/apr/30/national-health-service-bill.

49. This type of insurance is now being actively offered by major mortgage brokers, some of whom make the argument that those who can afford it should not risk their health relying on a less than comprehensive NHS.

50. LaingBuisson, *Private healthcare: Self-Pay UK market report*, 2020, www.laingbuisson.com/category/private-hospitals/.

51. LaingBuisson, *Private healthcare: Self-Pay UK market report*, 2021, 3rd edn., www.laingbuisson.com/shop/private-healthcare-self-pay-uk-market-report-3ed/.

52. As reported in Denis Campbell, 'NHS Waiting Times "driving people to turn to private treatment"', *Guardian*, 11 September 2017, www.theguardian.com/society/2017/sep/11/nhs-waiting-times-driving-people-to-turn-to-private-treatment.

53. See Jessica Murray, 'Fears of "two-tier" system as NHS waiting lists prompt more people to go private', *Guardian*, 27 October 2020, www.theguardian.

com/society/2020/oct/27/fears-of-two-tier-system-as-nhs-waiting-lists-prompt-more-people-to-go-private.

54. 'Out of pocket' expenditure figures available through the OECD 'Health Spending' dataset, data.oecd.org/healthres/health-spending.htm. 'Out of pocket' is a term that refers to health services purchased directly by private individuals, out of private savings.

55. Ibid. GDP figures available through the OECD 'Gross Domestic Product' dataset, data.oecd.org/gdp/gross-domestic-product-gdp.html.

56. £114 billion in 2018/19. Rachel Harker, *NHS expenditure*, UK Parliament research briefing, 17 January 2020, commonslibrary.parliament.uk/research-briefings/sn00724/#:~:text=In%202018%2F19%2C%20NHS%20England%20population%20and%20needs%2Dbased%20formula.

57. A move seen as so egregious that it prompted Nye Bevan to resign from the government. He had moved from minister of health to minister of labour and national service just months earlier – weakening the party ahead of a 1951 election it would go on to lose to Winston Churchill's Conservatives.

58. In the 1952 National Health Service Act. See, for example, House of Lords, *National Health Service Bill*, House of Lords, Hansard, May 1952, api.parliament.uk/historic-hansard/lords/1952/may/06/national-health-service-bill.

59. See Veronica Dale et al., *NHS dental charges and the effect of increases on access: An exploration*, University of York, the King's Fund/Prepare, 2021, www.york.ac.uk/media/healthsciences/images/research/prepare/NHS%20dental%20charges%20and%20the%20effect%20of%20increases%20on%20access%20-%20an%20exploration.pdf.

60. Stephen Armstrong, *The new poverty*, Verso, 2018.

61. John Curtice, 'Will Covid-19 change attitudes towards the welfare state?', *Progressive Review*, 27/1 (2020): 93–104.

62. Office for National Statistics, *NHS70: Marking 70 years of the National Health Service*, statistical briefing, 2018, www.ons.gov.uk/peoplepopulationandcommunity/healthandsocialcare/healthandwellbeing/articles/nhs70marking70yearsofthenationalhealthservice/2018-06-26.

63. British Heart Foundation. *Trends in coronary heart disease 1961-2011*, February 2011, www.bhf.org.uk/~/media/files/research/heart-statistics/bhf-trends-in-coronary-heart-disease01.pdf.

64. Macmillan Cancer Support, *Living after diagnosis: Median cancer survival times*, 2018, www.macmillan.org.uk/documents/aboutus/newsroom/livingaftercancermediancancersurvivaltimes.pdf.

65. The Richmond Group of Charities, *Just one thing after another*, 2018, richmondgroupofcharities.org.uk/sites/default/files/final_just_one_thing_after_another_report_-_singles.pdf.

66. Mai Stafford, Adam Steventon, Ruth Thorlby et al., *Understanding the health needs of people with multiple health conditions*, The Health Foundation, November 2018, www.health.org.uk/publications/understanding-the-health-care-needs-of-people-with-multiple-health-conditions.

67. Ibid. p. 1.

68. 16 years for women and 19 years for men – often, the whole of the average person's non-working life. Office for National Statistics, *Health State Life Expectancy, all ages, UK*, dataset, January 2021, www.ons.gov.uk/ peoplepopulationandcommunity/healthandsocialcare/healthandlife expectancies/datasets/healthstatelifeexpectancyallagesuk.

69. Predictably, during the pandemic, it went down fast. A study by Michael Marmot's Institute for Health Equity found that life expectancy fell by about a year in England (though disproportionately in some areas, normally where socio-economic deprivation is higher). Michael Marmot, Jessica Allen et al., *Build back fairer in Greater Manchester: Health equity and dignified lives*, Institute of Health Equity, June 2021, www.instituteofhealthequity.org/ resources-reports/build-back-fairer-in-greater-manchester-health-equity-and-dignified-lives/build-back-fairer-in-greater-manchester-main-report. pdf.

70. Michael Marmot et al., *Health equity in England: The Marmot Review 10 years on*, The Health Foundation/Institute of Health Equity, 2020, www. health.org.uk/publications/reports/the-marmot-review-10-years-on.

71. Veena S. Raleigh, 'Trends in life expectancy in EU and other OECD countries: Why are improvements slowing', *OECD Health Working Paper*, 108 (2019), https://doi.org/10.1787/223159ab-en.

72. Anne Case and Angus Deaton, 'Life expectancy in adulthood is falling for those without a BA degree, but as educational gaps have widened, racial gaps have narrowed', *PNAS*, 118/11 (2021), https://doi.org/10.1073/ pnas.2024777118.

73. From the website: www.nhsnewdeal.org/.

CHAPTER 1

1. Nick Thomas-Symonds MP replaced Diane Abbott as Shadow Home Secretary when Keir Starmer took over the Labour Party leadership.

2. Nicklaus Thomas-Symonds, *Nye: The political life of Aneurin Bevan*, I. B. Taurus, 2014, p. 2.

3. The Labour Party, *It's time for real change: The Labour Party manifesto 2019*, labour.org.uk/wp-content/uploads/2019/11/Real-Change-Labour-Manifesto-2019.pdf.

4. The Labour Party, '24 Hours to vote Labour and save the NHS', press release, 7 June 2017, labour.org.uk/press/24-hours-to-vote-labour-and-save-the-nhs/.

5. Team GB, 'Togetherness…', tweet, 5 July 2020, www.twitter.com/teamgb/ status/1279686703725326338.

6. Steve Richards, 'Don't laugh, politicians deserve pity not ridicule', *The Independent*, 1 August 2012, www.independent.co.uk/voices/commentators/ steve-richards/steve-richards-don-t-laugh-politicians-deserve-pity-not-ridicule-7999205.html.

7. For more on this bill see Nicholas Timmins, *Never again? The story of the Health and Social Care Act 2012*, The King's Fund, Institute for Government,

2012, www.kingsfund.org.uk/sites/default/files/field/field_publication_file/never-again-story-health-social-care-nicholas-timmins-jul12.pdf.

8. This was a cynical and dangerous language, and could justify its own section – but such critiques are well established and the focus here is what we can learn about leftist health discourse from the pandemic.

9. The Labour Party, 'Labour brands pay cut for the 225,000 NHS heroes in the Midlands the "ultimate insult"', press release, 18 March 2021, www.labour.org.uk/press/labour-brands-pay-cut-for-over-225000-nhs-heroes-in-the-midlands-the-ultimate-insult/.

10. Liberal Democrats, '1% pay rise is an insult to our NHS heroes says Lib Dems', press release, 1 March 2021, www.cheltlibdems.org.uk/give_nhs_heroes_a_pay_rise.

11. Ben Glaze, 'NHS heroes take to the streets to demand a pay rise from Tory Ministers', The Mirror, 11 September 2020, www.mirror.co.uk/news/politics/nhs-heroes-take-streets-demand-22663431.

12. Samantha Batt-Rawden, 'We need to stop calling NHS staff heroes – for a very important reason', The Independent, 1 May 2021, www.independent.co.uk/voices/nhs-covid-stress-burnout-heroes-b1840683.html.

13. Available at Wilfred Owen, 'Dulce et Decorum Est', 2021 [1920], Poetry Foundation, www.poetryfoundation.org/poems/46560/dulce-et-decorum-est.

14. YouGov, The NHS vs. European healthcare, tracker, 2021, www.yougov.co.uk/topics/travel/trackers/the-nhs-vs-european-healthcare.

15. Ibid. The rest either thought it was about the same (27 per cent) or don't know (19 per cent).

16. Eric C. Schneider et al., Mirror, mirror 2017: International comparison reflects flaws and opportunities for better U.S. health care, Commonwealth Fund, 2017, interactives.commonwealthfund.org/2017/uly/mirror-mirror/.

17. Our third place ranking on administrative efficiency will cause snide smiles among any healthcare workers reading – I have yet to meet anyone within the NHS who considers its administration efficient.

18. The 2021 follow-up to the rankings saw the UK slide to fourth place. This was put down to the impact of Covid-19, which impacted access to care and care processes.

19. At best, it sometimes sneaks into the middle of the pack.

20. Melina Arnold et al., 'Progress in cancer survival, mortality, and incidence in seven high-income countries 1995-2014 (ICBP SURVMARK-2): A population-based study', The Lancet, 20/11 (2019): 1493–1505, www.thelancet.com/journals/lanonc/article/PIIS1470-2045(19)30456-5/fulltext.

21. Irene Papanicolas et al., 'Performance of UK National Health Service compared with other high income countries: observational study', British Medical Journal, 367/l6326 (2019), www.bmj.com/content/367/bmj.l6326.

22. Rates of death from conditions that shouldn't prove fatal, with best practice healthcare in place. Christopher Murray et al., 'Healthcare access and quality index based on mortality from causes amenable to personal health care in

195 countries and territories, 1990 – 2015: A novel analysis from the global burden of disease study 2015', *The Lancet*, 390/10091 (July 2017): 231–266.

23. Russell Viney et al., 'Deaths in young people aged 0-24 years in the UK Compared with the EU15+ countries, 1970-2008: Analysis of the WHO Mortality Database', *The Lancet*, 384/9946 (2014): 880–892, www.thelancet. com/journals/lancet/article/PIIS0140-6736(14)60485-2/fulltext.

24. OECD, *Health at a glance: Europe 2016*, 2017, www.oecd.org/health/health-systems/Health-at-a-Glance-EUROPE-2016-Briefing-Note-UNITED%20 KINGDOM.pdf.

25. OECD, *United Kingdom: Raising standards*, 2016, read.oecd-ilibrary.org/ social-issues-migration-health/oecd-reviews-of-health-care-quality-united-kingdom-2016_9789264239487-en#page29.

26. Annabel Denham, 'Covid-19 has exposed the faults within the broken NHS System', *City A.M.*, 1 October 2020, www.cityam.com/ our-broken-nhs-system-needs-replacing/.

27. See Kristian Niemietz, 'Viral myths: Why we risk learning the wrong lessons from the pandemic', *Institute of Economic Affairs*, 9 February 2021, iea.org. uk/wp-content/uploads/2016/12/Niemietz-NHS-Interactive.pdf. For a wider account of the author's arguments see Kristian Niemietz, *Universal healthcare without the NHS*, Institute of Economic Affairs, 2016, iea.org.uk/ wp-content/uploads/2016/12/Niemietz-NHS-Interactive.pdf.

28. TaxPayers' Alliance, 'We need to find a new way to pay for healthcare', 22 January 2015, www.taxpayersalliance.com/we_need_to_find_a_new_way_ to_pay_for_healthcare.

29. Benedict Spence, 'The NHS is the closest thing we have to a religion – and that's why it must be privatised', *The Independent*, 7 February 2017, www. independent.co.uk/voices/nhs-crisis-jeremy-hunt-health-service-religion-privatise-save-it-a7567056.html; Fraser Coppin, 'The Big Debate: We need to privatise the NHS', *The Badger*, 1 March 2017, thebadgeronline. com/2017/03/big-debate-need-privatise-nhs/; Elizabeth Truss, 'The NHS is wrong to demonise privatisation', *The Telegraph*, 4 June 2008, www. telegraph.co.uk/comment/personal-view/3559102/The-NHS-is-foolish-to-demonise-privatisation.html.

30. Martin Gorsky, '"Searching for the people in charge": Appraising the 1983 Griffiths NHS Management Inquiry', *Medical History*, 57/1 (2013): 87–107.

31. Richard Lewis, 'Thirty years on, the Griffiths report makes interesting reading', *Health Service Journal*, 21 July 2014, www.hsj.co.uk/ future-of-nhs-leadership/thirty-years-on-the-griffiths-report-makes-interesting-reading/5072885.article.

32. Paul Joyce, 'Governmentality and risk: Setting priorities in the new NHS', *Sociology of Health and Illness*, 23/5 (2001): 594–614, onlinelibrary.wiley. com/doi/pdf/10.1111/1467-9566.00267.

33. Alternatively, they could reduce the cost of delivering care to those patients.

34. Integration would later be championed again by one of Labour's health advisors, Simon Stevens, upon becoming chief executive of the NHS in England (2014-2021). For some, the Johnson government's championing of

integration has associated it with privatisation, but conceptually it remains a potential collaboration-focused alternative to competition and markets.

35. 10 Downing Street Archives, *Speech by the Prime Minister Tony Blair about the NHS*, speech, 2017, web.archive.org/web/20080609053134/http://www.pm.gov.uk/output/Page1089.asp.

36. Polly Toynbee, 'NHS: The Blair years', *British Medical Journal*, 334/7602 (2001): 1030–1031, www.ncbi.nlm.nih.gov/pmc/articles/PMC1871752/.

37. NHS funding as a per cent of GDP had stagnated for several years under John Major and dropped slightly in the year before Blair was elected. It then rose from around 4.5 per cent to over 7.5 per cent during the Blair and Brown premierships. This is a much faster funding increase than seen in any other period of the NHS's history.

38. Documented in Toynbee, 'NHS: The Blair years'.

39. Robert Francis QC, *Report of the Mid Staffordshire HS Foundation Trust Public Inquiry*, 2013, assets.publishing.service.gov.uk/government/uploads/system/uploads/attachment_data/file/279124/0947.pdf.

40. Qtd in Kiran Stacey, 'Cameron defends "efficiency" drive', *Financial Times*, 8 May 2021, www.ft.com/content/8b5333ce-9939-11e1-948a-00144feabdc0.

41. Slightly unfairly, given that his role as an official was to implement the policy – but the design and direction was decided by politicians and ministers.

42. Institute for Fiscal Studies, *UK health spending*, 8 November 2019, https://ifs.org.uk/uploads/R165-UK-health-spending2.pdf.

43. NHS Confederation and NHS Providers, *A reckoning: the continuing cost of Covid-19*, 2 September 2021, https://nhsproviders.org/resource-library/briefings/a-reckoning-the-continuing-cost-of-covid-19

44. A pilot hosted by the World Economic Forum, and on which I was a member of the England team.

45. Chris Thomas, *Resilient health and care*, Institute of Public Policy Research, July 2020, www.ippr.org/files/2020-07/resilient-health-and-care-july20.pdf.

46. Ibid, p. 13.

47. OECD, *Hospital Beds*, dataset, 2020, data.oecd.org/healtheqt/hospital-beds.htm.

48. A. Bagust, 'Dynamics of bed use in accommodating emergency admissions: Stochastic simulation model', *British Medical Journal*, 319/7203 (2013): 155–158, emj.bmj.com/ content/21/5/575.long.

49. Chris Thomas, *Resilient health and care*.

50. Including bad flu seasons.

51. The Organisation for Economic Co-operation and Development – an international organisation with membership from the 'advanced economies'. Amongst other things, it provides data that shows how the UK performs against countries with broadly similar economic power – though, realistically, the UK remains a bigger economy that the vast majority of members. OECD, *Nurses*, dataset, 2020, data.oecd.org/healthres/nurses.htm; OECD, *Doctors*, dataset, 2019, data.oecd.org/healthres/doctors.htm.

52. OECD, *Long-Term care workforce: Caring for the ageing population with dignity*, 2017, www.oecd.org/health/health-systems/long-term-care-workforce.htm.

53. As per 2019, Office for National Statistics, *Employment in the UK: August 2019*, 2019, www.ons.gov.uk/employmentandlabourmarket/peopleinwork/employmentandemployeetypes/bulletins/employmentintheuk/august2019#:~:text=Download%20this%20chart,-Image%20.csv%20.xls&text=Estimates%20for%20April%20to%20June,year%20to%20reach%2024.11%20million.

54. NHS Confederation, *System under strain*, 30 April 2018, www.nhsconfed.org/sites/default/files/media/System-under-strain-report_0.pdf.

55. The Institute for Health Metrics and Evaluation, *Global burden of disease*, 2021, https://vizhub.healthdata.org/gbd-compare/.

56. British Heart Foundation. *Heart Failure: A blueprint for change*, 2021. www.bhf.org.uk/-/media/files/health-intelligence/heart-failure-a-blueprint-for-change.pdf?la=en&rev=f89dedb7c933452e8086cc063ff98c26&hash=98E3BEADD6A46974EF0AAD86044B8DC5314F4E2B.

57. A campaign idea most regularly found in Unite the Union.

58. See NHS Bill Now, *The bill*, www.nhsbillnow.org/the-bill/.

59. Chris Thomas, Harry Quilter-Pinner and Prashant Verma, *The innovation lottery*, Institute for Public Policy Research, 2020, www.ippr.org/files/2020-06/the-innovation-lottery-june20.pdf.

60. Ibid.

61. Taken from David Oliver, 'The pandemic has delivered clinical service innovations worth keeping', *British Medical Journal*, 373 (2020), https://doi.org/10.1136/bmj.n1306.

62. Wellcome Collection. *Medics, migration and the NHS*, 2018, https://wellcomecollection.org/articles/WyjPPScAALyZnoX7.

63. Bellinda Finlayson et al., 'Mind the gap: the extent of the NHS nursing shortage', *British Medical Journal*, 325/7363 (2002), doi: 10.1136/bmj.325.7363.538.

64. James Buchan et al., *Falling short*, The Health Foundation, November 2019, www.health.org.uk/publications/reports/falling-short-the-nhs-workforce-challenge.

65. See Rachel Worsley, 'We know the public love the NHS, but do they think it is a good employer', *The King's Fund*, 18 November 2019, www.kingsfund.org.uk/blog/2019/11/do-public-think-nhs-good-employer.

66. After the announcement and before the implementation of a 3 per cent pay rise for NHS workers covering 2021/2.

67. These figures vary due to the multitude way of calculating the figure. For this method, see Chris Thomas, 'Unjustifiable snub to exclude nurses and carers from pay boost, says IPPR', press release, Institute for Public Policy Research, 2020.

68. ITV, 'Revealed: Nurses forced to use food banks as Covid financial pressures drive many to brink of quitting', 17 December 2020, www.itv.com/

news/2020-12-17/revealed-nurses-forced-to-use-food-banks-as-covid-and-financial-pressures-drive-many-to-brink-of-quitting.

69. Hanna Wheatley, *Still no homes for nurses*, New Economics Foundation, 2019, neweconomics.org/uploads/files/StillNoHomes_May2019.pdf.

70. Parth Patel and Chris Thomas, *Recover, reward, renew: A post-pandemic plan for the healthcare workforce*, Institute of Public Policy Research, March 2021, www.ippr.org/research/publications/recover-reward-renew.

71. NHS Digital, *NHS workforce statistics*, NHS Digital, 2021. Available at: digital.nhs.uk/data-and-information/publications/statistical/nhsworkforce-statistics.

72. Mind, 'Two in five GPs have a mental health problem', 2018, www.mind.org.uk/news-campaigns/news/two-in-five-gps-have-a-mental-health-problem/.

73. Clare Gerada, 'Doctors and Suicide', *British Journal of General Practice*, 68/669 (2018): 168–169, bjgp.org/content/68/669/168#ref-2.

74. Lisa Elliott, Jonathon Tan and Sarah Norris, *The mental health of doctors: A systematic literature review*, Beyond Blue, 2010, das.bluestaronline.com.au/api/BEYONDBLUE/document?token=BL/0823

75. National Audit Office, *Discharging older patients from hospital*, Department of Health, 2016, www.nao.org.uk/report/discharging-older-patients-from-hospital/.

76. Thomas, *Resilient health and care*.

77. As a country average and over the course of a year. There will naturally be some oscillation – and having capacity to deal with that is the whole point.

78. Sometimes called an 'asset-based approach'.

79. Macmillan et al., *Improving the cancer journey: More than the sum of its parts, second report from a five-year evaluation by Edinburgh Napier University*, 30 September 2020, www.macmillan.org.uk/_images/Glasgow-improving-cancer-journey-programme-full-evaluation-2017_tcm9-324593.pdf.

80. For instance, Rebecca Thomas, 'Spending on Community Services cut by £300m', *Health Service Journal*, 19 July 2018, Hsj.co.uk/finance-and-efficiency/spending-on-community-services-cut-by-300m/7022954.article. See also Chris Thomas, 'Hitting the poorest worst? How public health cuts have been experienced in England's most deprived communities', *Institute of Public Policy Research*, 5 November 2011, IPPR.org/blog/public-health-cuts.

81. Indicatively, the creation of the NHS created an immediate shortage of 54,000 nurses – just through immediate increase in health provision.

82. Roberta Bivins, *The Windrush Generation and the NHS: By the Numbers*, People's History of the NHS, 2019, peopleshistorynhs.org/the-windrush-generation-and-the-nhs-by-the-numbers/.

83. Emma Jones and Stephanie Snow, 'Immigration and the National Health Service: Putting history to the forefront', *History and Policy*, 8 March 20211, www.historyandpolicy.org/policy-papers/papers/immigration-and-the-national-health-service-putting-history-to-the-forefron.

84. Emma Pitchforth, Michael Anderson, Chris Thomas et al., *Sustainability and resilience in the English health system*, London School of Economics, Partnership for Health System Sustainability and Resilience, www.3.weforum.org/docs/WEF_PHSSR_England_Report.pdf.

85. Matt Hancock, *NHS EI CNO Bulletin*, 2021, www.linkedin.com/pulse/ secretary-state-blog-international-nurse-recruitment-matt-hancock/.

86. Jonathan Ashworth, *Jonathan Ashworth Labour Party conference speech*, 28 September 2018, keepournhspublic.com/ashworth-conference-speech/.

87. MedAct, *Patients not passports: Challenging healthcare charging in the NHS*, October 2020, www.medact.org/wp-content/uploads/2020/10/ Patients-Not-Passports-Challenging-healthcare-charging-in-the-NHS-October-2020-Update.pdf

88. James Kirkup and Robert Winnett, 'Theresa May interview: "We're going to give illegal immigrants a really hostile reception"', *The Telegraph*, www.telegraph.co.uk/news/0/theresa-may-interview-going-give-illegal-migrants-really-hostile/.

89. World Health Organisation, *Health workforce*, www.who.int/health-topics/ health-workforce#tab=tab_1.

90. My analysis of the NHS England, *Cancer patient experience survey*, 2020, www.england.nhs.uk/statistics/statistical-work-areas/cancer-patient-experience-survey/.

91. NHS England, *NHS workforce race equality standard*, 2019, www.england. nhs.uk/wp-content/uploads/2020/01/wres-2019-data-report.pdf.

92. Ibid, p. 13.

93. Patel and Thomas, *Recovery, reward, renew*.

94. Cabinet Office, *Race disparity audit: Summary findings from the Ethnicity Facts and Figures website*, October 2017, www.ethnicity-facts-figures.service. gov.uk/static/race-disparity-audit-summary-findings.pdf.

95. Ibid.

96. Marie Curie, *Palliative and end of life care for Black, Asian and Minority Ethnic Groups in the UK*, 2013, www.mariecurie.org.uk/globalassets/media/ documents/policy/policy-publications/june-2013/palliative-and-end-of-life-care-for-black-asian-and-minority-ethnic-groups-in-the-uk.pdf.

CHAPTER 2

1. D. W. Lewis, 'What was wrong with Tiny Tim', *American Journal of Diseases of Children*, 146/12 (1992): 1403–1407, pubmed.ncbi.nlm.nih.gov/1340779/.

2. R. W. Chesney, 'Environmental factors in Tiny Tim's near-fatal illness' *Archives of Paediatric and Adolescent Medicine*, 166/3 (2012): 271–275, doi:10.1001/archpediatrics.2011.852.

3. At this point in history modern treatments for TB would not have been available, contextualising the author's choice further.

4. Ibid.

5. Quoted in David Olusanga and Melanie Backe-Hansen, *A house through time*, Picador, 2020.

6. Ministry of Housing, Communities and Local Government, *English housing survey: Headline report*, 2020, www.wassets.publishing.service.gov.uk/government/uploads/system/uploads/attachment_data/file/945013/2019-20_EHS_Headline_Report.pdf.

7. Department for Business, Energy and Industrial Strategy, *Annual fuel poverty statistics in England*, 2020, 30 April 2020, www.assets.publishing.service.gov.uk/government/uploads/system/uploads/attachment_data/file/882404/annual-fuel-poverty-statistics-report-2020-2018-data.pdf.

8. Lucie Middlemiss and Ross Gilard, 'Fuel poverty from the bottom-up: Characterising household energy vulnerability through the lived experience of fuel poor', *Energy Research and Social Science*, 6/1 (2015): 146–154, www.reader.elsevier.com/reader/sd/pii/S2214629615000213?token=87E3C870E732CDCF8CD91B414B8759F99423085F2A868B24EED205A738FAB30DD5514EBA15225B4C5F67AC16108696A3.

9. Sorcha Daly, *Later life in the UK*, Institute of Health Equity, University College London, 2016, www.institutehealthequity.blogspot.com/.

10. See Emer O'Connell, 'How your body copes with cold weather', *Public Health England*, 21 October 2019, https://publichealthmatters.blog.gov.uk/2019/01/16/how-your-body-copes-with-cold-weather/.

11. Ministry of Housing, Communities and Local Government, English Housing Survey, Headline Report, 2018–2019, www.assets.publishing.service.gov.uk/government/uploads/system/uploads/attachment_data/file/860076/2018-19_EHS_Headline_Report.pdf.

12. Ibid.

13. Gangtani Pnnumam et al., 'Socioeconomic Deprivation and Notification Rates for Tuberculosis in London during 1982-91', *British Medical Journal*, 350 (1995): 963–966, www.ncbi.nlm.nih.gov/pmc/articles/PMC2549356/pdf/bmj00588-0017.pdf.

14. For primary evidence see: Khansa Ahmad et al., 'Association of poor housing conditions with Covid-19 incidence and mortality across us counties', *Plos One*, 2020, https://doi.org/10.1371/journal.pone.0241327 N; J. A. Patel et al., 'Poverty, inequality and Covid-19: The forgotten vulnerable', *Public Health*, 183 (2020): 110–111, journals.plos.org/plosone/article?id=10.1371/journal.pone.0241327.

15. Rebecca Roberts-Hughes, *The case for space*, Royal Institute of British Architects, Homewise, 2011, www.brand-newhomes.co.uk/RIBA-Case-for-space-2011.pdf.

16. National Housing Federation, '1 in 7 people in England directly hit by the housing crisis', 2011, www.housing.org.uk/news-and-blogs/news/1-in-7-people-in-england-directly-hit-by-the-housing-crisis/.

17. I recognise these cannot be distinguished from class, but rather add a different, intersectional dynamic to experiences of health injustice.

18. D. D. Reid et al., 'Cardiorespiratory disease and diabetes among middle-aged male civil servants: a study of screening and intervention', *The Lancet*, 303/7854 (1974): 469–473, www.thelancet.com/journals/lancet/article/PIIS0140-6736(74)92783-4/fulltext.

19. Michael G. Marmot et al. 'Health inequalities among British Civil Servants; The Whitehall II Study', *The Lancet*, 337/8754 (1991): 1387–1393, www. thelancet.com/journals/lancet/article/PII0140-6736(91)93068-K/fulltext.

20. Equality and Human Rights Commission, *Is Britain fairer: Key facts and findings on ethnicity*, 2015, www.equalityhumanrights.com/sites/default/ files/is-britain-fairer-findings-factsheet-ethnicity.pdf; Institute for Government, *Why does ethnic diversity in the civil service matter?*, www. instituteforgovernment.org.uk/explainers/ethnicity-civil-service.

21. His half day off at Christmas is very hard won.

22. HM Government, *Good work: The Taylor review of modern working practices*, 2017, assets.publishing.service.gov.uk/government/uploads/ system/uploads/attachment_data/file/627671/good-work-taylor-review-modern-working-practices-rg.pdf.

23. Trade Union Congress, *Living on the margins: Black workers and casualisation*, 2015, www.tuc.org.uk/sites/default/files/LivingontheMargins. pdf.

24. M.E. Davies and E. Hoyt, 'A longtitudinal study of piece rate and health: Evidence and implications for workers in the US gig economy', *Public Health*, 180 (2020): 1–9, www.sciencedirect.com/science/article/pii/ S0033350619303415

25. Ursula Huws, Neil H. Spencer et al., *Work in the European gig economy: Research results from the UK, Sweden, Germany, Austria, The Netherlands, Switzerland, and Italy*, Foundation for European Progressive Studies (FEPS), 2017, uhra.herts.ac.uk/bitstream/handle/2299/19922/Huws_U._Spencer_ N.H._Syrdal_D.S._Holt_K._2017_.pdf.

26. Back pain is often not taken seriously, but when measuring its consequences in terms of 'disability adjusted life years' – a measure that looks to account for quality of life, not just quantity – it has a larger aggregate impact on health in England than lung cancer or ischaemic heart disease. Nicholas Steel et al., 'Changes in health in the countries of the UK and 150 English Local Authority areas 1990–2016: a systematic analysis for the Global Burden of Disease Study 2016', *The Lancet*, 392/10158 (2018): 1647–1661, https://doi.org/10.1016/S0140-6736(18)32207-4.

27. Ibid.

28. Ibid.

29. Department for Business, Energy, and Industrial Strategy, *The characteristics of those in the gig economy*, 2018, www.gov.uk/government/publications/ gig-economy-research.

30. Elena Cottini, 'Health at Work and Low Pay: A European Perspective', *The Manchester School*, 80/1 (2011): 75–98, onlinelibrary.wiley.com/doi/abs /10.1111/j.1467-9957.2011.02250; Elena Cottini, and Claudio Lucifora, *Inequalities at work: Job quality, health and low pay in European workplaces*, GINI Discussion Paper 86, August 2013, http://archive.uva-aias.net/ uploaded_files/publications/86-4-3-4.pdf.

31. Tracy Shildrick et al., *The low-pay, no-pay cycle*, Joseph Rowntree Foundation, November 2010, www.basw.co.uk/system/files/resources/basw_123014-5_0.pdf.

32. And the striver/shirker binary it relied on. Indicatively, see Patrick Wintour, 'Welfare reforms: We will make work pay, says George Osborne', *Guardian*, 2 April 2013, www.theguardian.com/politics/2013/apr/02/george-osborne-work-welfare-tax.

33. Andrew Smith, Emma Wadsworth and Christina Shaw, *Ethnicity, work characteristics, stress and health*, Cardiff University and Queen Mary, University of London, Health & Safety Executive, 2005, www.hse.gov.uk/research/rrpdf/rr308.pdf.

34. HM Government, *Race in the workplace: The McGregor-Smith Review*, Department for Business, Energy and Industrial Strategy, February 2017, assets.publishing.service.gov.uk/government/uploads/system/uploads/attachment_data/file/594336/race-in-workplace-mcgregor-smith-review.pdf.

35. And was roundly rejected by the Thatcher government.

36. Michael Marmot et al., *Fair society healthy lives (the Marmot review)*, February 2012, www.instituteofhealthequity.org/resources-reports/fair-society-healthy-lives-the-marmot-review.

37. HM Government, *Ministry of Health Act 1919*, 1919, www.legislation.gov.uk/ukpga/Geo5/9-10/21/enacted.

38. Department of Health and Social Care, *Prevention is better than cure: Our vision to help you live well for longer*, white paper, 2018, www.gov.uk/government/publications/prevention-is-better-than-cure-our-vision-to-help-you-live-well-for-longer.

39. Boris Johnson, 'Face-it, it's all your own fat fault', *The Telegraph*, 27 May 2004, www.telegraph.co.uk/politics/0/face-fat-fault/.

40. Patrick Wintour and Colin Blackstock, 'Let the poor smoke, says health secretary', *Guardian*, 9 June 2004, www.theguardian.com/uk/2004/jun/09/smoking.politics.

41. Ben Bradley MP, 'Tweet 6 September 2020, 8.05pm', *Twitter*, twitter.com/bbradley_mans/status/1302684380327030790.

42. Dolly R.Z. Theis and Martin White, 'Is Obesity Policy in England Fit for Purpose? Analysis of Government Strategies and Policies, 1992-2020', *The Milbank Quarterly*, 99/1 (2021): 126–170, https://doi.org/10.1111/1468-0009.12498.

43. All author's analysis of Public Health England, *Local authority health profiles*, data, 2021, fingertips.phe.org.uk/profile/health-profiles.

44. Joint Strategic Needs Assessment Blackpool, *Housing and homelessness*, 2020, www.blackpooljsna.org.uk/People-and-Places/Wider-determinants-of-health/Housing.aspx#HousingQualityinBlackpool.

45. Public Health England, *Local authority health profiles: Blackpool*, 2021, fingertips.phe.org.uk/profile/health-profiles/data#page/13/gid/1938132696/pat/6/par/E12000002/ati/202/are/E06000009/cid/4.

46. escholarship.org/content/qt4sz4s617/qt4sz4s617.pdf.

47. Ibid.

48. Arguably NHS provision also stops before the end of the pathway. The hospice movement delivers a great deal of end of life and palliative care, but it is funded by the voluntary sector, and does not have nearly enough beds to provide good quality care for all. That means the NHS covers three of the seven steps in my model pathway.

49. The King's Fund, *Making the case for public health interventions*, 2014, www.kingsfund.org.uk/audio-video/public-health-spending-roi.

50. S. Martin et al., *Is an ounce of prevention worth a pound of cure?*, University of York, 2019, www.york.ac.uk/media/che/documents/papers/researchpapers/CHERP166_Impact_Public_Health_Mortality_Morbidity.pdf.

51. Thomas, 'Hitting the poorest worst?'.

52. Chris Thomas, Anna Round and Sarah Longlands, *Levelling-up health for Prosperity*, Institute for Public Policy Research, 2020, www.ippr.org/research/publications/levelling-up-health-for-prosperity

53. Chris Thomas, *Progress at last*, Institute for Public Policy Research, forthcoming.

54. Outside of certain exceptional circumstances.

55. Michael Marmot et al., *Fair Society, Healthy Lives*, 2010, www.parliament.uk/globalassets/documents/fair-society-healthy-lives-full-report.pdf.

56. Jo Bibby, *How do our education and skills influence our health?*, The Health Foundation, 2017, www.health.org.uk/infographics/how-do-our-education-and-skills-influence-our-health.

57. Department for Education, *Permanent and fixed-period exclusions in England*, data, 2020, explore-education-statistics.service.gov.uk/find-statistics/permanent-and-fixed-period-exclusions-in-england.

58. Ibid.

59. T. J. Ford et al., 'The relationship between exclusion from school and mental health: A secondary analysis of the British Child and Adolescent Mental Health Surveys, 2004-2007', University of Exeter, 2017, ore.exeter.ac.uk/repository/bitstream/handle/10871/28337/Psychological%20medicine%20revision%2023%20June%202017.pdf?sequence=1.

60. Zahra Bei et al., 'How do we progress racial justice in education', *Progressive Review*, 28/1 (2021), https://doi.org/10.1111/newe.12242.

61. Education Policy Institute, *Unexplained Pupil Exits from Schools: A Growing Problem?*, 2019, epi.org.uk/publications-and-research/unexplained-pupil-exits/.

62. Sally Weale, 'Attainment gap between poor pupils and their peers in England is widening', *Guardian*, 26 August 2020, www.theguardian.com/education/2020/aug/26/attainment-gap-between-poor-pupils-and-their-peers-widening.

63. Hilary Stewart et al., 'The cost of school holidays for children from low income families', *Childhood*, 25/4 (2018): 516–529, https://doi.org/10.1177/0907568218779130.

64. As also concluded by the Sutton Trust. See Rebecca Montacute, *Social Mobility and Covid-19*, Sutton Trust, 2020, www.suttontrust.com/wp-content/uploads/2020/04/COVID-19-and-Social-Mobility-1.pdf.

65. Rates available at Education and Skills Funding Agency, *Pupil Premium: Conditions of grant 2021 to 2022 for local authorities*, 2021, www.gov.uk/government/publications/pupil-premium-allocations-and-conditions-of-grant-2021-to-2022/pupil-premium-conditions-of-grant-2021-to-2022-for-local-authorities.

66. Luke Sibieta, *2020 Annual report on education spending in England*, Institute for Fiscal Studies, 18 September 2020, www.ifs.org.uk/publications/15025.

67. Independent Schools Council, *ISC annual census*, 7 May 2021, www.isc.co.uk/research/annual-census/.

68. Nicholas W. Papageorge and Kevin Thom, 'Genes education and labor market outcomes: Evidence from the Health and Retirement Study', *National Bureau of Economic Research*, 18/3 (2020): 1351–1399, https://doi.org/10.1093/jeea/jvz072.

69. That is not to say that private schools should continue – while outside the remit of the public health service, repurposing these assets for public use would be worthwhile from a health perspective.

70. Of course, it would not just be the children receiving the extra investment that benefit – there would be a knock-on positive effect for everyone.

71. Anna Ambrose and Harry Quilter-Pinner, *The new normal: The future of education after Covid-19*, Institute of Public Policy Research, October 2020, www.ippr.org/research/publications/the-new-normal.

72. Eva Orberle, 'Screen time and extracurricular activities as risk and protective factors for mental health in adolescence: a population-level study', *Journal of Preventative Medicine*, 141 (December 2020), https://doi.org/10.1016/j.ypmed.2020.106291.

73. Nicola Wright et al., 'Interplay between long-term vulnerability and new risk: Young adolescent and maternal mental health immediately before and during the COVID-19 pandemic', *JCPP Advances*, 1/1 (2021), https://doi.org/10.1177/0907568218779130.

74. Feeding Britain, *Ending hunger in the holidays*, 2017, feedingbritain.org/wp-content/uploads/2019/01/Ending_Hunger_in_the_Holiday_Report_Dec_2017-3.pdf.

75. Public Health England, *Obesity profile*, NHS Digital, 2021, digital.nhs.uk/services/national-child-measurement-programme/.

76. Corinna Hawkes et al., 'Smart food policies for obesity prevention', *The Lancet*, 345 (2015), http://repositorio.uchile.cl/bitstream/handle/2250/133565/Smart-food-policies-forobesity-prevention.pdf?sequence=1.

77. Dean Hochlaf and Chris Thomas, *The whole society approach*, Institute of Public Policy Research, 27 August 2020, www.ippr.org/research/publications/the-whole-society-approach.

78. Susan Lloyd, *Rose vouchers for fruit and veg – an evaluation report*, Lambeth Project Final Evaluation, 2017, www.alexandrarose.org.uk/Handlers/Download.ashx?IDMF=d22cf114-923d-4dec-84a2-22fbed94f7f7.

79. Paul Coleman et al., *Building a food system that works for everyone*, Institute of Public Policy Research, April 2021, www.ippr.org/research/publications/building-a-food-system-that-works-for-everyone.

80. Luke Murphy et al., *Fairness and opportunity*, Institute of Public Policy Research, July 2021, www.ippr.org/research/publications/fairness-and-opportunity.

81. Stuart Adam et al., *Social housing in England: A survey*, Institute for Fiscal Studies, November 2015, www.ifs.org.uk/uploads/publications/bns/BN178.pdf#page=9.

82. Trust for London, *London's poverty profile*, 2020, www.trustforlondon.org.uk/data/rent-affordability-borough/#:~:text=In%20every%20London%20borough%20the,gross%2Dmedian%20pay%20in%20London.

83. As per Clare et al., *No longer managing*, Institute of Public Policy Research, 2021, www.ippr.org/research/publications/no-longer-managing-the-rise-of-working-poverty-and-fixing-britain-s-broken-social-settlement.

84. Social Prosperity Network, *Social prosperity for the future: A proposal for universal basic services*, UCL Institute for Global Prosperity, 2017, www.ucl.ac.uk/bartlett/igp/sites/bartlett/files/universal_basic_services_-_the_institute_for_global_prosperity_.pdf.

85. Crisis, *Homelessness monitor*, 2019, www.crisis.org.uk/ending-homelessness/about-homelessness/#:~:text=There%20is%20no%20national%20figure,are%20homeless%20across%20the%20UK.&text=For%20the%20last%20five%20years,at%20the%20end%20of%202019.

86. Many of these with overlap with the kind of private rented sector homes that come with serious health hazards. HM Government, *Overcrowded households*, 2020, www.ethnicity-facts-figures.service.gov.uk/housing/housing-conditions/overcrowded-households/latest. This varies significantly by ethnicity, with 24 per cent of Bangladeshi households living in over-crowded homes, compared to 2 per cent of white British households.

87. Centre for Public Impact, *Eradicating homelessness in Finland: The housing first programme*, 2019, www.centreforpublicimpact.org/case-study/eradicating-homelessness-finland-housing-first-programme.

88. Ibid.

89. Lynne Chester and Alan Morris, 'A New Form of energy poverty is the hallmark of liberalised electricity sectors', *Australian Journal of Social Issues*, 46/4 (2016), https://doi.org/10.1002/j.1839-4655.2011.tb00228.x.

90. Office for National Statistics, *Exploring the UK Digital Divide*, 2019, statistical briefing, www.ons.gov.uk/peoplepopulationandcommunity/householdcharacteristics/homeinternetandsocialmediausage/articles/exploringtheuksdigitaldivide/2019-03-04.

91. Centre for Economic and Business Research, *The economic impact of basic digital skills and inclusion in the UK*, 2015, www.goodthingsfoundation.org/insights/economic-impact-basic-digital-skills/.

92. Joseph Rowntree Foundation, *How does money influence health?*, 2015, www.jrf.org.uk/report/how-does-money-influence-health.

93. Siobhan Palmer 'Homelessness a "major issue" for employers, new figures suggest', 2019, www.peoplemanagement.co.uk/news/articles/homelessness-a-major-issue-for-employers#gref

94. Joseph Rowntree Foundation, *UK Poverty 2019/20*, 2019, www.jrf.org.uk/file/54566/download?token=nBjYDICV&filetype=full-report.

95. Trussell Trust, 'Do working people need food banks', FAQ, 6 November 2019, www.trusselltrust.org/2019/11/06/working-people-at-food-banks/.

96. The Liberal Democrats, *But what is a skills wallet?*, 2019, www.libdems.org.uk/skills-wallet.

97. Kela, 'Results of Finland's basic income experiment: small employment effects, better perceived economic security and mental wellbeing', press release, 2020, www.kela.fi/web/en/news-archive/-/asset_publisher/lNo8GY2nIrZo/content/results-of-the-basic-income-experiment-small-employment-effects-better-perceived-economic-security-and-mental-wellbeing.

98. Kela, *Basic income experiment*, 2020, www.kela.fi/web/en/basic-income-experiment.

99. A. C. Logan et al., 'Golden Age of Medicine 2.0: Lifestyle Medicine and Planetary Health Prioritised' *Journal of Lifestyle Medicine*, 9/2 (2019): 75–91, www.ncbi.nlm.nih.gov/pmc/articles/PMC6894443/.

CHAPTER 3

1. It later emerged this was only true because they'd launched a massive campaign of free samples for doctors, just before the survey period.

2. Tracy A. Ruegg, 'Historical perspectives of the causation of lung cancer', *Global Quality of Nursing Research*, 2, www.ncbi.nlm.nih.gov/pmc/articles/PMC5342645/.

3. Robert Proctor, 'The History of the discovery of the cigarette-lung cancer link: evidentiary traditions, corporate denial, global toll', *Tobacco Control*, 21/2(2012), tobaccocontrol.bmj.com/content/21/2/87; Centers for Disease Control and Prevention, 'Achievements in public health, 1900-1999: Tobacco use – United States, 1900-1999', *Morbidity and Mortality Weekly Report*, 48/43 (1999), www.cdc.gov/mmwr/preview/mmwrhtml/mm4843a2.htm.

4. An ingenious cohort to choose because they are registered and can be easily followed up with.

5. Richard Doll et al., 'Mortality in relation to smoking: 50 years' observations on male British doctors', *British Medical Journal*, 328/7455 (2014); 1519, www.ncbi.nlm.nih.gov/pmc/articles/PMC437139/#ref11.

6. Action on Smoking and Health, *Key Dates in Tobacco Regulation 1962 – 2020*, 16 April 2020, ash.org.uk/wp-content/uploads/2020/04/Key-Dates.pdf.

7. British American Tobacco, *The global market*, 2020, www.bat.com/group/sites/UK__9D9KCY.nsf/vwPagesWebLive/DO9DCKFM#:~:text=The%20most%20recent%20estimates%20for,19%25%20of%20the%20world's%20

population; The Tobacco Atlas, *Consumption*, 2016, tobaccoatlas. org/topic/consumption/#:~:text=About%205.7%20trillion%20 (5%2C700%2C000%2C000%2C000)%20cigarettes%20were%20smoked%20 worldwide%20in%202016.

8. Tobacco Manufacturers Association, *Fast facts*, http://the-tma.org.uk/ fast-facts/; Tobacco Manufacturers Association, *Tobacco industry in the UK*, http://resource.download.wjec.co.uk.s3.amazonaws.com/vtc/2014- 15/15_07_Economics/pdf/cbac/uned7/25.%20Tobacco%20Industry%20 Data.pdf.

9. Nicholas Lyett, 'Imperial Brands – Dividend Increased', Hargreaves Lansdown, financial results, 18 May 2021, www.hl.co.uk/shares/ share-research/202105/imperial-brands-dividend-increase.

10. BAT, *Building the enterprise of the future: Annual report and form 20-f 2020*, 2020, www.bat.com/annualreport.

11. Philip Morris International, *Together. forward: 2020 annual report*, 2021, www.pmi.com/resources/docs/default-source/investor_relation/pmi_2020_ annualreport.pdf?sfvrsn=402b8eb4_2.

12. Office for National Statistics, *Adult smoking habits in the UK: 2019*, statistical bulletin, 2020, www.ons.gov.uk/peoplepopulationandcommunity/ healthandsocialcare/healthandlifeexpectancies/bulletins/adultsmoking habitsingreatbritain/2019#:~:text=In%202019%2C%20the%20proportion %20of,falling%20smoking%20prevalence%20since%202011; Public Health England, *Smoking and tobacco: Applying all our health*, 16 June 2020, www.gov.uk/government/publications/smoking-and- tobacco-applying-all-our-health/smoking-and-tobacco-applying- all-our-health.

13. Office for National Statistics, *Coronavirus (COVID-19): 2020 in charts*, 2020, www.ons.gov.uk/peoplepopulationandcommunity/healthand socialcare/conditionsanddiseases/articles/coronaviruscovid192020 incharts/2020-12-18.

14. National Health Service, *What are the health risks of smoking?*, www.nhs.uk/ common-health-questions/lifestyle/what-are-the-health-risks-of-smoking/.

15. I.e., deaths that could be prevented with the right intervention.

16. Sanjay Agrawal, *Health inequalities and tobacco*, Royal College of Physicians, 2020, www.rcplondon.ac.uk/news/health-inequalities-and- tobacco#:~:text=In%20the%20UK%2C%20tobacco%20use,and%20 the%20most%20deprived%20communities.&text=Currently%20a%20 quarter%20of%20a,due%20to%20expenditure%20on%20tobacco.

17. CDC (undated), *Smoking and tobacco use*, fact sheet, www.cdc.gov/tobacco/ data_statistics/fact_sheets/fast_facts/index.htm.

18. Sarah E. Jackson et al. 'Moderators of changes in smoking, drinking and quitting behaviour associated with the first COVID-19 lockdown in England', *Addiction*, 25 August 2021, https://doi.org/10.1111/add.15656.

19. Dereck Yach and Douglas Bettcher, 'Globalisation of tobacco industry influence and new global responses', *Tobacco Control*, 9/2 (2000): 206–216, tobaccocontrol.bmj.com/content/9/2/206.

20. Gianna Gayle Herrera Amul et al., 'A systematic review of tobacco industry tactics in Southeast Asia: Lessons for other low-and-middle-income regions', *International Journal of Health Policy and Management*, 10/6 (2021): 1–14, www.ijhpm.com/article_3834_3be135653f75d1a0228559cfdaad2103.pdf.

21. Luk Joossens, 'Vietnam: Smuggling adds Value', *Tobacco Control*, 12/2 (2003): 119–120, tobaccocontrol.bmj.com/content/12/2/119.

22. J. Collin et al., 'Complicity in contraband: British American tobacco and cigarette smuggling in Asia', *Tobacco Control*, 13/2 (2004), tobaccocontrol. bmj.com/content/12/2/119.

23. And also, beyond it, which sit outside my reflections here.

24. The focus on companies that cost the NHS money is another example of NHS-centrism limiting the scope and scale of the progressive public health mainstream.

25. The Labour Party, *Medicines for the many: Public health before private profit*, 2019, labour.org.uk/wp-content/uploads/2019/09/Medicines-For-The-Many.pdf.

26. Imperial College London, 'Obesity has doubled since 1980, major global analysis of risk factors reveals', 4 February 2011, www.imperial. ac.uk/news/96402/obesity-doubled-since-1980-major-global/#:~: text=BMI%3A,cent%20for%20women%20in%201980.&text=The%20 UK%20has%20the%20sixth,around%2027%20kg%2Fm2; Hochlaf and Thomas, *The whole society approach*.

27. Anne Case and Angus Deaton, *Deaths of Despair and the Future of Capitalism*, Princeton University Press, 2020.

28. GambleAware, 'Nearly half of all people with gambling disorder have not accessed treatment or support according to in-depth research into the demand for treatment of gambling harms', press release, 2020, www. begambleaware.org/sites/default/files/2020-12/2020-05-19-treatment-needs-gap-analysis-press-release.pdf.

29. Beveridge won a Berwick-upon-Tweed by-election in 1944, only to be defeated in the 1945 general election and subsequently made a peer.

30. Margaret Jones and Rodney Lowe, *From Beveridge to Blair*, Manchester University Press, 2002.

31. William Beveridge, *Social insurance and allied services*, HM Government, November 1942, www.ncbi.nlm.nih.gov/pmc/articles/PMC2560775/pdf/10916922.pdf.

32. Indeed, it is often noted that the NHS is a treatment not a whole health service – which is the basis for the Universal Public Health Service outlined in Chapter 2.

33. Average retirement age is 64 years old, and average healthy life expectancy is 63 years old. ONS, *Healthy state life expectancies, UK: 2017-2019*, 2021, www. ons.gov.uk/peoplepopulationandcommunity/healthandsocialcare/health andlifeexpectancies/bulletins/healthstatelifeexpectanciesuk/2017to2019.

34. David Cameron, *PM Speech on Wellbeing*, 25 November 2010, www.gov.uk/government/speeches/pm-speech-on-wellbeing.

35. David Cameron, *Transforming the British Economy: Coalition strategy for economic growth*, 2010, www.gov.uk/government/speeches/transforming-the-british-economy-coalition-strategy-for-economic-growth.

36. Institute for Fiscal Studies, *Recent cuts to public spending*, 2015 www.ifs.org.uk/tools_and_resources/fiscal_facts/public_spending_survey/cuts_to_public_spending.

37. Harry Quilter-Pinner, *The end of austerity*, Institute of Public Policy Research, 18 April 2019, www.ippr.org/blog/austerity-there-is-an-alternative-and-the-uk-can-afford-to-deliver-it.

38. Kate Raworth, *Doughnut economics: Seven ways to think like a 21st century economist*, Penguin Random House, 2017. See Chapter One, available at doughnuteconomics.org/tools-and-stories/18; see also Kate Raworth, 'Why it's time for Doughnut Economics'. *Progressive Review*, 24/3 (2017): 216–222, onlinelibrary.wiley.com/doi/abs/10.1111/newe.12058.

39. Kate Raworth, 'Seven ways to think like a 21st century economist', *OpenDemocracy*, 5 April 2017, www.opendemocracy.net/en/transformation/seven-ways-to-think-like-21st-century-economist/.

40. Robert F. Kennedy, *Remarks at the University of Kansas*, 18 March 1968, www.jfklibrary.org/learn/about-jfk/the-kennedy-family/robert-f-kennedy/robert-f-kennedy-speeches/remarks-at-the-university-of-kansas-march-18-1968.

41. Jacqueline McGlade et al., 'Towards a sustainable wellbeing economy', April 2019 www.researchgate.net/profile/Paul-Sutton/publication/332233189_Towards_a_sustainable_economy/links/5cacb5b3458515cd2b0beofc/Towards-a-sustainable-economy.pdf; B. F. Giannetti et al. 'A review of limitations of GDP and alternative indices to monitor human wellbeing and to manage eco-system functionality', *Journal of Cleaner Production*, 87/1(2015): 11–25, www.advancesincleanerproduction.net/papers/journals/2014/2014_jcp.pdf; Catherine Colebook, *Measuring what matters: Improving the indicators of economic performance*, Institute of Public Policy Research, 2018, www.ippr.org/publications/measuring-what-matters.

42. At least in the short-term – and almost all governments working to a five-year election cycle significantly over-value the short-term.

43. E. Stamatakis et al., 'Overweight and obesity trends from 1974 to 2003 in English children: what is the role of socioeconomic factors?', *Archives of Disease in Childhood*, 90/10 (2004), adc.bmj.com/content/90/10/999; Public Health England, *Obesity profile for England*, fingertips.phe.org.uk/profile/national-child-measurement-programme/data.

44. Matthew Limb, 'Deaths from alcohol hit record high during 2020, show figures', *British Medical Journal*, 327 (2021), https://doi.org/10.1136/bmj.n317.

45. House of Lords Select Committee on the Social and Economic Impact of the Gambling Industry, *Gambling harm – Time for action*, 2020, https://publications.parliament.uk/pa/ld5801/ldselect/ldgamb/79/79.pdf.

46. Office for National Statistics, *Human health and social work activities (£M):CP*, dataset, 2020, www.ons.gov.uk/economy/gross domesticproductgdp/timeseries/kkn7/bb.

47. There is some evidence from the Covid-19 pandemic that suggests the UK measures GDP in a way that is particularly susceptible to this problem. Office for National Statistics, *Comparisons of GDP during the Coronavirus (COVID-19) pandemic*, 2021, www.ons.gov.uk/economy/grossdomesticproductgdp/articles/internationalcomparisonsofgdpduring thecoronaviruscovid19pandemic/2021-02-01.

48. Simon Stevens, *Simon Stevens speech to Institute of Directors Annual Convention*, 7 October 2015, www.england.nhs.uk/2015/10/directors-convention/.

49. Hochlaf and Thomas, *The whole society approach.*

50. See for instance, the work of Gillian Pascall – including Gillian Pascall, *Social policy: A feminist analysis*, Tavistock Press, 1986; Gillian Pascall, *Social policy: A new feminist analysis*, Routledge, 1997; and Gillian Pascall, *Gender equality in the welfare state*, Policy Press, 2012.

51. See for example Jameel Hampton, *Disability and the welfare state in Britain: Changes in perception and policy 1948-1979*, Policy Press, 2016.

52. Johnathan Watkins et al., 'Effects of health and social care spending constraints on mortality in England: A time trend analysis', *BMJ Open*, 2017, bmjopen.bmj.com/content/7/11/e017722.citation-tools; For a similar figure from a different method, see also: Hochlaf et al., *Ending the blame game*, Institute of Public Policy Research, 2019, www.ippr.org/research/publications/ending-the-blame-game.

53. Clare Bambra et al., *Health for wealth*, Northern Health and Science Alliance,2018, www.thenhsa.co.uk/app/uploads/2018/11/NHSA-REPORT-FINAL.pdf.

54. Chris Thomas et al., *Levelling-up health for prosperity*, Institute of Public Policy Research, 2021, www.ippr.org/research/publications/levelling-up-health-for-prosperity.

55. 2019 estimates. See Statista, 'Gross value added (GVA) of agriculture in the United Kingdom (UK) from 2003 to 2019', data, 2021, www.statista.com/statistics/315804/agriculture-gross-value-added-in-the-united-kingdom-uk/.

56. Public Health England, 'Third year of industry progress to reduce sugar published', 2020, www.gov.uk/government/news/third-year-of-industry-progress-to-reduce-sugar-published.

57. Mark Petticrew, 'Dark nudges and sludge in big alcohol: Behavioural economics, cognitive biases, and alcohol industry corporate social responsibility', *The Milbank Quarterly*, 98/4 (2020): 1290–1328, online library.wiley.com/doi/full/10.1111/1468-0009.12475.

58. Ibid.

59. Drinkaware, *Alcohol and cancer*, www.resourcesorg.co.uk/assets/pdfs/Alcohol-and-cancer.pdf.

60. As per D. M. Parkin, 'Cancers attributable to consumption of alcohol in the UK in 2010' *British Journal of Cancer*, 105/.Suppl 2 (2011): S14–18, 10.1038/bjc.2011.476.

61. With exceptions for some high-sugar drinks that may arguably be healthy (e.g., fresh orange juice).

62. HM Revenue and Customs, *Soft drinks industry levy statistics commentary 2020*, 2021, www.gov.uk/government/statistics/soft-drinks-industry-levy-statistics/soft-drinks-industry-levy-statistics-commentary-2020#:~:text=Soft%20Drinks%20Industry%20Levy%20Receipts,-Headlines&text=Total%20SDIL%20receipts%20for%20financial,not%20due%20until%20July%202018.

63. See Vera Zakharov et al., 'Refreshing investment in children's health: Using the Sugary Drinks Tax to improve healthy food access in schools', School Food Matters, 2020, www.schoolfoodmatters.org/sites/default/files/Refreshing-Investment-in-Childrens-Health.pdf.

64. Action on Sugar, *Sugar reduction: Report on progress between 2015 and 2019*, 2020, www.actiononsugar.org/news-centre/sugar-in-the-news/2020/2020-stories/sugar-reduction-report-on-progress-between-2015-and-2019.html.

65. Cherry Law, 'An analysis of the stock market reaction to the announcements of the UK Soft Drinks Industry Levy', *Economics and Human Biology*, 38/1 (2020), www.sciencedirect.com/science/article/pii/S1570677X19302096?via%3Dihub.

66. E. Martos, *Assessment of the impact of a public health product tax: Final report*, World Health Organisation, 2015, www.euro.who.int/__data/assets/pdf_file/0008/332882/assessment-impact-PH-tax-report.pdf.

67. Emma Smith et al., 'Should we tax unhealthy food and drink?', *Proceedings of the Nutritional Society* 77/3 (2019): 314–320, www.ncbi.nlm.nih.gov/pmc/articles/PMC5912513/.

68. Office for National Statistics, *Gender pay gap in the UK: 2020*, 2020, www.ons.gov.uk/employmentandlabourmarket/peopleinwork/earningsandworkinghours/bulletins/genderpaygapintheuk/2020.

69. Clara Guibourg and Eleanor Lawrie, 'Gender pay gap grows at hundreds of big firms', *BBC*, 20 February 2019, www.bbc.co.uk/news/business-47252848#:~:text=The%20BBC%20looked%20at%20a,and%20the%20middle%2Dranking%20man.&text=Of%20those%201%2C146%20companies%2C%20the,improvement%20from%209.7%25%20last%20year.

70. Jonathan Platt, 'Unequal depression for equal work? How the wage gap explains gendered disparities in mood disorders', *Social Science and Medicine*, 149 (2016): 1–8, www.sciencedirect.com/science/article/abs/pii/S0277953615302616.

71. Chartered Insurance Institute, *Securing the financial future of the next generation*, Insuring Women's Futures, 2018, www.cii.co.uk/media/9224351/iwf_momentsthatmatter_full.pdf.

72. Office for National Statistics, *Human Capital Estimates in the UK: 2004 to 2018*, 2019, www.ons.gov.uk/peoplepopulationandcommunity/wellbeing/articles/humancapitalestimates/2004to2018#human-capital-by-sex.

73. British Heart Foundation, *How has the smoking ban changed our health?*, 2017, www.bhf.org.uk/informationsupport/heart-matters-magazine/news/smoking-ban; See also Michelle Sims et al., 'Short term impact of smoke-free legislation in England: retrospective analysis of hospital admissions for myocardial infarction', *British Medical Journal*, 340 (2010), https://doi.org/10.1136/bmj.c2161.

74. Action on Smoking and Health, *Smokefree: The First Ten Years*, 2017, ash.org.uk/wp-content/uploads/2017/06/170107-Smokefree-the-first-ten-years-FINAL.pdf.

75. See James Meadway, 'Creating the digital commons after COVID-19', *OpenDemocracy*, 2020, www.opendemocracy.net/en/oureconomy/creating-digital-commons-after-covid-19/.

76. Nominet, *Digital Access for All launches to solve problem of digital exclusion*, press release, 2019, www.nominet.uk/digital-access-for-all-launches-to-help-solve-problem-of-digital-exclusion/.

77. For example, Harisa Mardiana, 'The impact of teenagers' digital literacy on the use of social media', *The 3rd International Conference of Advance & Scientific Innovation*, 20 June 2020, www.researchgate.net/publication/345783914_The_Impact_of_Teenagers'_Digital_Literacy_on_the_Use_of_Social_Media.

78. See Sonia Livingstone, 'Developing social media literacy: how children learn to interpret risky opportunities on social network sites', *Communications*, 39/3 (2014): 283–303, http://eprints.lse.ac.uk/62129/1/Developing%20social%20media%20literacy.pdf.

79. Department for Education, *Bullying in England April 2013 to March 2018*, 2018, assets.publishing.service.gov.uk/government/uploads/system/uploads/attachment_data/file/754959/Bullying_in_England_2013-2018.pdf

80. Gwen Schurgin O'Keeffe and Kathleen Clarke-Pearson, 'The impact of social media on children, adolescents, and families', *Pediatrics*, 127/4 (2011): 800–804, www.cooperativa.cl/noticias/site/artic/20110329/asocfile/20110329173752/reporte_facebook.PDF.

81. Ofcom, ICO, *Internet users' concerns about and experience of potential online harms*, 2019, www.ofcom.org.uk/__data/assets/pdf_file/0028/149068/online-harms-chart-pack.pdf.

82. S. Boniface, C. Thomas, J. Vohra et al., 'Underage adolescents' reactions to adverts for beer and spirit brands and associations with higher risk drinking and susceptibility to drink: a cross-sectional study in the UK', *Alcohol and Alcoholism*, agab018 (2021), https://doi.org/10.1093/alcalc/agab018; Nathan Critchlow et al., 'Awareness of marketing for high fat, salt or sugar foods and the association with higher weekly consumption among adolescents: a rejoinder to the UK government's consultations on marketing regulation', *Public Health Nutrition*, 23/14 (2020): 2637–2646, www.stir.ac.uk/research/hub/publication/1500476; Nathan Critchlow et al., 'Social media, higher risk consumption, and brand identification', *Addiction Research and Theory*, 27/6 (2021): 515–526, www.stir.ac.uk/research/hub/publication/1074907;

Chris Thomas et al., *Under pressure*, Cancer Research UK, 2020, www.cancerresearchuk.org/sites/default/files/under_pressure.pdf.

83. See Rhianna Schmunk, 'B.C. pub company partially at fault for drunk-driving crash, judge rules', *CBC*, 10 March 2017, www.cbc.ca/news/canada/british-columbia/pub-liability-drunk-driver-1.4020142.

84. See Center for Democracy and Technology, *Overview of the NetzDG Network Enforcement Law*, 2017, https://cdt.org/insights/overview-of-the-netzdg-network-enforcement-law/.

85. Alcohol control is often an area where public health policies are most advanced, if only thanks for the long impact of the temperance movement. In Britain, it emerged from the 'gin craze'.

86. Government Offices of Sweden, *Swedish alcohol retailing monopoly (Systembolaget Aktiebolag)*, www.government.se/government-agencies/swedish-alcohol-retailing-monopoly--systembolaget-aktiebolag/.

87. Tea Olsen, 'Explaining the strong support for the Swedish alcohol retail monopoly', *Institute of Alcohol Studies*, 24 May 2019, www.ias.org.uk/2019/05/24/explaining-the-strong-support-for-the-swedish-alcohol-retail-monopoly/.

88. Tim Stockwell et al., 'Estimating the public health impact of disbanding a government alcohol monopoly: Application of new methods to the case of Sweden', *BMC Public Health*, 18/1400 (2018), bmcpublichealth.biomedcentral.com/articles/10.1186/s12889-018-6312-x. Corroborating evidence from 2010. See Thor Norström et al., 'Potential consequences of replacing a retail alcohol monopoly with a private licence system: results from Sweden', *Addiction*, 105/12 (2010): 2113–2119.

89. Medieakademin, *Förtroendebarometern*, 2019, medieakademin.se/wp-content/uploads/2019/03/F%C3%B6rtroendebarometern-2019-1.pdf.

90. Robin Room, 'Alcohol monopolies', *Shaap*, 12 February 2021, www.shaap.org.uk/blog/332-alcohol-monopolies.html.

91. Helping to explain why this chapter has not advocated for any public health bans.

92. Robin Room and Jenny C. Örnberg, 'Government monopoly as an instrument for public health and welfare: Lessons for cannabis from experience with alcohol monopolies', *International Journal of Drug Policy*, 74 (2019), doi: 10.1016/j.drugpo.2019.10.008.

93. For example Jonathan P. Caulkins and Beau Kilmer 'The US as an example of how *not* to legalize marijuana', *Addiction*, 111/12 (2016): 2095–2096, https://onlinelibrary.wiley.com/doi/10.1111/add.13498; Rachel Barry and Stanton Glantz, 'Marijuana regulatory frameworks in four US states: an analysis against a public health standard', *American Journal of Public Health*, 108/7 (2018): 914–923, www.ncbi.nlm.nih.gov/pmc/articles/PMC5993386/; Rachel Barry and Stanton Glantz, 'A public health framework for legalized retail marijuana based on the US experience: avoiding a new tobacco industry', *Plos Medicine*, 13/9 (2016), https://journals.plos.org/plosmedicine/article?id=10.1371/journal.pmed.1002131.

94. Kojo Koram, *Cannabis and capitalism*, Common Wealth, 2019, www.common-wealth.co.uk/interactive-digital-projects/cannabis-and-capitalism.

95. Estimate from Buzzfeed Amanda Chicago Lewis, 'America's whites-only weed boom', *Buzzfeed News*, 16 March 2020, www.buzzfeednews.com/article/amandachicagolewis/americas-white-only-weed-boom.

96. James Meadaway, *Creating a digital commons*, Institute of Public Policy Research, 2020, www.ippr.org/files/2020-08/creating-a-digital-commons-august20.pdf; British Academy and The Royal Society, *Data management and use: governance in the 21st century*, June 2017, https://royalsociety.org/-/media/policy/projects/data-governance/data-management-governance.pdf.

97. European Parliament, *Is data the new oil?*, 2020, www.europarl.europa.eu/RegData/etudes/BRIE/2020/646117/EPRS_BRI(2020)646117_EN.pdf .

CHAPTER 4

1. Parth Patel et al., *State of health and care*, Institute of Public Policy Research, 2021, www.ippr.org/files/2021-03/state-of-health-and-care-mar21.pdf.

2. HM Government, *National Assistance Act*, 1948, www.legislation.gov.uk/ukpga/Geo6/11-12/29.

3. The King's Fund 'The origins and development of social care', undated, www.kingsfund.org.uk/sites/default/files/Securing_Good_Care_Chapter_1.pdf.

4. Stewart Player and Allyson Pollock, 'Long-term care: from public responsibility to private good', *Critical Social Policy*, 21/2 (2001): 231–255.

5. The same Roy Griffiths who reviewed the NHS in Chapter One.

6. Roy Griffiths, *Community care: Agenda for action*, HMSO, 1988.

7. Ray Jones, 'A Journey through the Years: Ageing and Social Care', *Ageing Horizons*, 6 (2007): 42–51.

8. Player and Pollock, 'Long-term care'; p. 235.

9. Jones, Ray, 'A Journey through the Years'.

10. Not enacted until 1993.

11. HM Government, *National Health Service and Community Care Act 1990*, 1990, www.legislation.gov.uk/ukpga/1990/19/contents

12. Player and Pollock, 'Long-term care'. https://allysonpollock.com/wp-content/uploads/2013/04/CriticalSocialPolicy_2001_Player_LongTermCare.pdf

13. Bob Hudson, 'The unsuccessful privatisation of social care: why it matters and how to curb it', *London School of Economics*, 4 April 2016, blogs.lse.ac.uk/politicsandpolicy/why-social-care-privatisation-is-unsuccessful/?utm_content=buffer4a900&utm_medium=social&utm_source=twitter.com&utm_campaign=buffer.

14. Grace Blakeley and Harry Quilter-Pinner, *Who cares? The financialisaton of adult social care*, Institute of Public Policy Research, 2019, www.ippr.org/files/2019-09/who-cares-financialisation-in-social-care-2-.pdf.

15. Ibid, p. 6.

16. Hudson, 'The unsuccessful privatisation of social care'.

17. At the time of writing, one is in administration.

18. Blakeley and Quilter-Pinner, *Who cares?*.

19. Joe Dromey and Dean Hochlaf, *Fair care: A workforce strategy for social care*, Institute for Public Policy Research, 25 November 2018, www.ippr.org/research/publications/fair-care.

20. Care Quality Commission, *The state of adult social care services 2014 to 2017: Findings from the CQCs initial programme of comprehensive inspections in adult social care*, 2018, www.cqc.org.uk/sites/default/files/20170703_ASC_end_of_programme_FINAL2.pdf; Unison, 'Employers in the care sector are hiding behind complex and incomplete pay slips to break wage laws', press release, 2018, www.unison.org.uk/news/2018/04/employers-care-sector-hiding-behind-complex-incomplete-pay-slips-break-wage-laws/; Susan C. Eaton, 'Beyond "unloving care": linking human resource management and patient care quality in nursing homes', *The International Journal of Human Resource Management*, 11/3 (2000): 591–616.

21. Care Quality Commission, *The state of adult social care services 2014 to 2017*.

22. Care Quality Commission, *The state of health care and adult social care in England 2019/20*, 2020, www.cqc.org.uk/sites/default/files/20201016_stateofcare1920_fullreport.pdf.

23. Ara Darzi, *Better health and care for all*, Institute of Public Policy Research, 2018, www.ippr.org/files/2018-06/better-health-and-care-for-all-june2018.pdf.

24. The King's Fund, *How serious are the pressures in social care?*, 2015, www.kingsfund.org.uk/projects/verdict/how-serious-are-pressures-social-care.

25. Christopher Thomas, *Health inequalities: Time to talk*, Macmillan Cancer Support, 2019, www.macmillan.org.uk/assets/health-inequalities-paper-april-2019.pdf.

26. Tania Burchardt et al., 'The Conservatives' record on adult social care', London School of Economics Centre for Analysis of Social Exclusion, 3 November 2020, https://sticerd.lse.ac.uk/CASE/_NEW/PUBLICATIONS/abstract/?index=7525.

27. Age UK, 'The number of older people with some unmet need for care now stands at 1.5 million', 9 November 2019, www.ageuk.org.uk/latest-press/articles/2019/november/the-number-of-older-people-with-some-unmet-need-for-care-now-stands-at-1.5-million/.

28. The Health Foundation, *Social care for adults aged 18-64*, April 2020, www.health.org.uk/publications/reports/social-care-for-adults-aged-18-64.

29. Independent Age, *Free personal care: How to eliminate catastrophic care costs*, 2021, independent-age-assets.s3.eu-west-1.amazonaws.com/s3fs-public/2019-04/Final%20Report_Web_0.pdf.

30. Ibid.

31. Excluding certain costs, like hotel costs.

32. Chris Thomas, 'The "make do and mend" health service: Solving the NHS's Capital Crisis', *Institute of Public Policy Research*, 2019, www.ippr.org/research/publications/the-make-do-and-mend-health-service.

33. Ibid.

34. National Audit Office, *Investigation into the collapse of Carillion*, 2019, www.nao.org.uk/report/investigation-into-the-governments-handling-of-the-collapse-of-carillion/.

35. See Graeme Wearden, 'The rise and fall of Southern Cross', *Guardian*, 1 June 2011, www.theguardian.com/business/2011/jun/01/rise-and-fall-of-southern-cross.

36. Nina Lakhani, 'Southern Cross collapse leaves elderly care in Limbo', *The Independent*, 23 October 2011, www.independent.co.uk/life-style/health-and-families/health-news/southern-cross-collapse-leaves-elderly-care-in-limbo-2312648.html.

37. Care Quality Commission, *Whitchurch care home: Inspection report*, 15 February 2019, https://api.cqc.org.uk/public/v1/reports/64ce2d22-5d83-441e-9a64-1ed6f83adb47?20200129163919.

38. Ibid., p. 3.

39. Name changed to protect anonymity.

40. Skills for Care, *The state of the adult social care sector and workforce in England*, 2020, www.skillsforcare.org.uk/adult-social-care-workforce-data/Workforce-intelligence/documents/State-of-the-adult-social-care-sector/The-state-of-the-adult-social-care-sector-and-workforce-2020.pdf.

41. Ibid.

42. Ibid.

43. Stewart Sutherland, *With respect to old age: A report by the Royal Commission on Long Term Care*, HM Government, 1999, www.scie-socialcareonline.org.uk/with-respect-to-old-age-a-report-by-the-royal-commission-on-long-term-care/r/a11G00000017xMvIAI.

44. Despite the fact they were tripling the NHS's budget, and the health of social care is key to how effectively the NHS can use its own funding.

45. Mark Ivory, *Tony Blair: The Social Care Legacy*, Community Care, 2007, www.communitycare.co.uk/2007/05/09/tony-blair-the-social-care-legacy/.

46. Luke Clements, Louisa Harding Edgar and Allyson M Pollock, 'Why we need a National Care Service – and how to Build One', *Tribune*, 22 June 2020, tribunemag.co.uk/2020/06/towards-a-national-care-service-2.

47. GMB Union, *5 Key Asks: Social Care*, 2021, www.gmb.org.uk/sites/default/files/CARE_GOPUBLIC_2020.pdf.

48. We Own It, *Why we need a National Care Service*, 2021, weownit.org.uk/blog/why-we-need-national-care-service.

49. The Scottish context is slightly different. They did introduce free personal care in 2002. Scottish National Party, 'How is the SNP improving social care services?', 2021, www.snp.org/policies/pb-how-is-the-snp-improving-social-care-services/.

50. Dean Hochlaf and Harry Quilter-Pinner, *Social care: Free at the point of need*, Institute of Public Policy Research, May 2019, www.ippr.org/files/2019-05/social-care-free-at-the-point-of-need-may-19.pdf.

51. Independent Age, 'Three-quarters of adults in England back free personal care for over-65s, says charity', press release, 6 September 2018, www.independentage.org/news-media/press-releases/three-quarters-of-adults-england-back-free-personal-care-for-over-65s.

52. Richard Sloggett and Harry Quilter-Pinner, *Care after Coronavirus: An emerging consensus*, Institute of Public Policy Research, Policy Exchange, May 2020, www.ippr.org/blog/ippr-policy-exchange-social-care-polling.

53. Patel et al., *State of health and care*.

54. CHPI, *Plugging the Leaks in the UK care home industry*, 2019, chpi.org.uk/wp-content/uploads/2019/11/CHPI-PluggingTheLeaks-Nov19-FINAL.pdf.

55. Particularly, disabled people – with the debate often unbalanced in focusing on people over 65 years old.

56. Michel Foucault, *Madness and civilization: A history of insanity in the Age of Reason*, Pantheon Books, 1965.

57. Leonard Cheshire, *Adult Social Care April 2018*, 2018, www.leonardcheshire.org/sites/default/files/2019-03/social_care_briefing_-_leonard_cheshire.docx.

58. Christina R. Victor, 'Loneliness in care homes: a neglected area of research?', *Ageing Health*, 8/6 (2012), www.futuremedicine.com/doi/abs/10.2217/ahe.12.65.

59. NHS England, '1.18i – Social Isolation: percentage of adult social care users who have as much social contact as they would like', survey data, 2016, data.england.nhs.uk/dataset/phe-indicator-90280/resource/9d56da41-f81c-4262-97b3-edaa1abab411.

60. Independent Age, *Free personal care: Insights from Scotland*, 2020, independent-age-assets.s3.eu-west-1.amazonaws.com/s3fs-public/2020-10/Report_Final.pdf?5pNaZ4vjvNoJt4YGK2Bctq4DOnK9_fp2=.

61. Ibid.

62. Social Care Future, *Talking about a brighter social care future*, 2019, socialcarefuture.files.wordpress.com/2019/10/ic-scf-report-2019-h-web-final-111119.pdf.

63. See Reclaiming the Future Alliance, *Independent living for the future*, 2019, dpac.uk.net/2019/04/a-national-independent-living-support-service/.

64. Jack Hunter and Martina Orvolic. *End of life care in England*, Institute of Public Policy Research, May 2018, www.ippr.org/files/2018-05/end-of-life-care-in-england-may18.pdf.

65. Chris Thomas, *Community first social care*, Institute for Public Policy Research, 23 August 2021, www.ippr.org/research/publications/community-first-social-care.

66. Care Quality Commission, *The state of adult social care services: 2014 to 2017*.

67. Maurice McLeod and Chris Thomas, 'Racism is not a culture war toy – it's a fact of life in Tory Britain', *Tribune*, 22 June 2021, tribunemag.co.uk/2021/06/racism-is-not-a-culture-war-toy-its-a-fact-of-life-in-britain.

68. CADTH, 'Dementia Villages: Innovative Residential Care for People with Dementia', 2019, 178, www.cadth.ca/sites/default/files/hs-eh/eh0071-dementia-villages.pdf, pp. 2–28.

69. See Centre for Policy on Ageing, *Foresight Future of An Ageing Population – International Case Studies*, 2016, www.cpa.org.uk/information/reviews/

CPA-International-Case-Study-4-Housing-and-Dementia-Care-in-the-Netherlands.pdf.

70. CADTH, 'Dementia Villages'.

71. Sandy Ransom, *Eden alternative: The Texas Project*, IQILTHC Series Report 2000–2004, 2000, digital.library.txstate.edu/bitstream/handle/10877/4087/fulltext.pdf?sequence=1&isAllowed=y.

72. Daniel Button and Sarah Bedford, *Ownership in social care: Why it matters and what can be done*, New Economics Foundation, 2020, neweconomics.org/2020/01/ownership-in-social-care.

73. Simon Borkin, *Platform co-operatives – solving the capital conundrum*, Nesta, 2019, media.nesta.org.uk/documents/Nesta_Platform_Report_FINAL-WEB_b1qZGj7.pdf.

74. Institute of Public Policy Research, *Prosperity and justice*, www.ippr.org/files/2018-08/1535639099_prosperity-and-justice-ippr-2018.pdf.

75. Ibid.

76. Harry Quilter-Pinner, *Ethical Care: A bold reform agenda for adult social care*, Institute of Public Policy Research, 2019, www.ippr.org/research/publications/ethical-care.

77. Skills for Care, *The state of the adult social care sector and workforce in England*.

78. Marcus Johns, *10 Years of Austerity: Eroding Resilience in the North*, Institute of Public Policy Research, 2020, www.ippr.org/research/publications/10-years-of-austerity.

79. Quilter-Pinner, *Ethical care*.

80. ONS, *Household satellite account, UK: 2015 and 2016*, 2018, www.ons.gov.uk/economy/nationalaccounts/satelliteaccounts/articles/householdsatelliteaccounts/2015and2016estimates.

81. Carers UK, *Juggling work and unpaid care: A growing issue*, 2019, www.carersuk.org/images/News_and_campaigns/Juggling_work_and_unpaid_care_report_final_0119_WEB.pdf.

82. Ibid.

83. New Policy Institute, *Informal carers and poverty in the UK: An analysis of the Family Resources Survey*, 2019, npi.org.uk/files/2114/6411/1359/Carers_and_poverty_in_the_UK_-_full_report.pdf.

84. Raphael Wittenberg, 'Projects of demand for and costs of social care for older people in England, 2010 to 2030, under current and alternative funding systems', *PSSRU*, December 2011, http://eprints.lse.ac.uk/40720/1/2811-2.pdf.

85. Andrea Budnick et al., 'Informal caregivers during the COVID-19 pandemic perceive additional burden', *BMC Health Services Research*, 21/353 (2021), bmchealthservres.biomedcentral.com/articles/10.1186/s12913-021-06359-7.

86. Carers UK, *Caring behind closed doors: Six months on*, 2020, www.carersuk.org/images/News_and_campaigns/Caring_Behind_Closed_Doors_Oct20.pdf.

87. Author's analysis of Office for National Statistics, *Household Satellite Account, UK*, dataset, 2018, www.ons.gov.uk/economy/nationalaccounts/satelliteaccounts/compendium/householdsatelliteaccounts/2005to2014/relateddata.

88. See Chris Thomas, *The state of end of life care*, Institute of Public Policy Research, 2021, www.ippr.org/files/2021-04/end-of-life-care-april21.pdf.

89. Carers UK, *The case for care leave*, 2013, www.carersuk.org/ for-professionals/policy/policy-library?task=download&file=policy_file&id=218.

CHAPTER 5

1. Global Health Security Index, *Global Health Security Index*, 2019, www.ghsindex.org/wp-content/uploads/2019/10/2019-Global-Health-Security-Index.pdf.

2. Johns Hopkins University, *Coronavirus mortality*, dataset, 2021, coronavirus.jhu.edu/data/mortality.

3. In the time between writing and publication, the ability of affluent countries to monopolise the Covid-19 vaccine could change this picture significantly.

4. The sudden name change suggesting a very deliberate change in emphasis (i.e., from protection to security).

5. Matt Hancock, *Reinvigorating our system for international health*, speech, 26 January 2021, www.gov.uk/government/speeches/reinvigorating-our-system-for-international-health.

6. Kate Jones et al., 'Trends in emerging infectious diseases', *Nature*, 451 (2008): 990–993, www.nature.com/articles/nature06536/.

7. Ibid.

8. For instance, HM Government, *Life sciences vision*, 2021, assets.publishing.service.gov.uk/government/uploads/system/uploads/attachment_data/file/1000030/life-sciences-vision.pdf.

9. Katherine Smith et al., 'Global rise in human infectious disease outbreaks', *Journal of the Royal Society*, 6 December 2014, royalsocietypublishing.org/doi/full/10.1098/rsif.2014.0950.

10. World Economic Forum, 'Outbreak Readiness and Business Impact: Protecting Lives and Livelihoods across the Global Economy', white paper, 2019, www.3.weforum.org/docs/WEF%20HGHI_Outbreak_Readiness_Business_Impact.pdf.

11. Ibid.

12. Ibid, p. 5.

13. World Health Organisation, *Crimean Congo Haemorrhagic Fever*, 2013, www.who.int/en/news-room/fact-sheets/detail/crimean-congo-haemorrhagic-fever.

14. World Health Organisation, *Ebola Virus Disease*, 2021, www.who.int/news-room/fact-sheets/detail/ebola-virus-disease,

15. World Health Organisation, *Marburg Virus Disease*, 2018, www.who.int/news-room/fact-sheets/detail/marburg-virus-disease.

16. World Health Organisation, *Lassa Fever*, www.who.int/health-topics/lassa-fever#tab=tab_1.

17. World Health organisation, *Nipah Virus*, 2019, www.who.int/news-room/fact-sheets/detail/nipah-virus.

18. Ibid.

19. Various, 'The threat of pandemic influenza: are we ready? Workshop summary', *The National Archives*, www.ncbi.nlm.nih.gov/books/NBK22148/.

20. Jenny Hope, 'How £300 million was squandered on swine flu jabs that we didn't need', *The Daily Mail*, 7 April 2010, www.dailymail.co.uk/news/article-1263975/Swine-flu--300m-squandered-jabs-didnt-need.html.

21. Gabriele Neumann and Yoshihiro Kawaoka, 'Predicting the Next Influenza Pandemics', *Journal of Infectious Diseases*, 219/S1 (2019): S14–20, www.ncbi.nlm.nih.gov/pmc/articles/PMC6452319/.

22. Zhi-Ping Zhong et al., 'Glacier ice archives fifteen-thousand-year-old viruses', *BioRxiv*, 7 January 2020, www.biorxiv.org/content/10.1101/2020.01.03.894675v1.

23. Elisa Stella et al., 'Permaforst dynamics and the risk of anthrax transmission: a modelling study', *Scientific Reports*, 10, /16460 (2020), www.nature.com/articles/s41598-020-72440-6; www.biorxiv.org/content/10.1101/486290v1.

24. Enoch J. Abbey et al., 'The Global Health Security Index is not predictive of coronavirus pandemic response among Organisation for Economic Cooperation and Development countries', *Plos One*, 7 October 2020, https://doi.org/10.1371/journal.pone.0239398.

25. And vitally, understood outside of the excellent but rather isolated world of global health academia.

26. Stockholm Resilience Centre, *The nine planetary boundaries*, www.stockholmresilience.org/research/planetary-boundaries/planetary-boundaries/about-the-research/the-nine-planetary-boundaries.html.

27. Jonathan Patz, 'A human disease indicator for the effects of recent global climate change', *PNAS*, 99/20 (2020): 12506-12508, www.pnas.org/content/99/20/12506; Jonathan Patz et al., *Climate change and infectious diseases*, World Health Organisation, 2013, www.who.int/globalchange/publications/climatechangechap6.pdf; Jonathan Patz et al., 'Global climate change and emerging infectious diseases', *JAMA*, 275/3 (1996): 217–223, pubmed.ncbi.nlm.nih.gov/8604175/.

28. S. W. Lindsay and W. J. Martens, W.J., 'Malaria in the African highlands: Past, present and future', *Bulletin of the World Health Organization*, 76/1 (1998): 33–45.

29. J. Hartman et al., 'Climate suitability for stable malaria transmission in Zimbabwe under different climate change scenarios', *Global Change & Human Health*, 3/1 (2002): 42–53.

30. Jeffrey Shaman et al., 'Using a dynamic hydrology model to predict mosquito abundances in flood and swamp water', *Emerging Infectious Diseases*, 8/1 (2002): 6–13.

31. Paul R. Epstein, 'West Nile virus and the climate', *Journal of Urban Health*, 78/2 (20021): 367–371.

32. William Checkley et al., 'Effect of El Niño and ambient temperature on hospital admissions for diarrhoeal diseases in Peruvian children', *The Lancet*, 355/9202 (2000): 442–450.

33. Dana A. Fockset al., 'A simulation model of the epidemiology of urban dengue fever: Literature analysis, model development, preliminary validation, and samples of simulation results', *American Journal of Tropical Medicine and Hygiene*, 53/5 (1995): 489–506.

34. Joachim Rocklöv and Robert Dubrow, 'Climate change: an enduring challenge for vector-borne disease prevention and control', *Nature Immunology*, 21/5 (2020): 479-483, www.nature.com/articles/s41590-020-0648-y.

35. United Nations, *Climate change key findings*, www.un.org/en/climatechange/science/key-findings.

36. World Meteorological Organization, *WMO Greenhouse Gas Bulletin*, 14 (November 2018), library.wmo.int/doc_num.php?explnum_id=5455.

37. Jeff Tollefson, 'COVID curbed carbon emissions in 2020 – but not by much', *Nature*, 15 January 2021, www.nature.com/articles/d41586-021-00090-3.

38. William J. Ripple et al., 'World scientists' warning to humanity: a second notice', *BioScience*, 67/12 (2017): 1026–1028, academic.oup.com/bioscience/article/67/12/1026/4605229.

39. Daniel W. O'Neill et al., 'A Good life for all within planetary boundaries', *Nature Sustainability*, 1 (2018): 88–95, www.nature.com/articles/s41893-018-0021-4; Laurie Laybourn-Langton et al., *This is a crisis*, Institute of Public Policy Research, 2019, www.ippr.org/research/publications/age-of-environmental-breakdown.

40. Toph Allen, 'Global Hotspots and correlates of emerging zoonotic diseases', *Nature Communications*, 8/1124 (2017), www.nature.com/articles/s41467-017-00923-8; R. T. Corlett, *State of the tropics*, James Cooks University, www.jcu.edu.au/state-of-the-tropics/publications/2014-state-of-the-tropics-report; S. Nazrul Islam and John Winkel, 'Climate Change and Social Inequality', *DESA Working Paper*, 152 (2017), www.un.org/esa/desa/papers/2017/wp152_2017.pdf; United States Environmental Protection Agency, *International Climate Impacts*, 19 January 2017, 19january2017snapshot.epa.gov/climate-impacts/international-climate-impacts_.html.

41. P. Daszak et al., 'Anthropogenic environmental change and the emergence of infectious diseases in wildlife', *Act Tropica*, 78 (2001): 103-116.

42. Daszak, 'Anthropogenic environmental change and the emergence of infectious diseases in wildlife'.

43. Jason Rohr et al., 'Emerging human infectious diseases and the links to global food production', *Nature Sustainability*, 2 (2019): 445–456, www.nature.com/articles/s41893-019-0293-3.

44. Bryony A. Jones et al., 'Zoonosis emergence linked to agricultural intensification and environmental change', *Proceedings of the National*

Academy of Sciences USA, 110/21 (2013): 8399–8404, www.ncbi.nlm.nih.
gov/pmc/articles/PMC3666729/.

45. Jones, 'Zoonosis emergence linked to agricultural intensification and environmental change'.

46. Hannah Ritchie and Max Roser, *Land use*, Our World in Data, 2019, ourworldindata.org/land-use.

47. Ibid.

48. Max Roser, 'Two centuries of rapid global population growth will come to an end', *Our World in Data*, 2019, ourworldindata.org/world-population-growth-past-future.

49. Kate E. Jones et al., 'Global Trends in Emerging Infectious Diseases', *Nature*, 451/7181 (2008): 990–993, www.ncbi.nlm.nih.gov/pmc/articles/PMC5960580/.

50. United Nations, *World Urbanization Prospects 2018*, dataset, 2018, population.un.org/wup/.

51. Hannah Ritchie and Max Roser, *Urbanization*, Our World in Data, 2019, ourworldindata.org/urbanization.

52. Creighton Connolly et al 'Extended urbanisation and the spatialities of infectious disease: Demographic change, infrastructure and governance', *Urban Studies*, 58/2 (2021): 245–263, 254, https://journals.sagepub.com/doi/pdf/10.1177/0042098020910873.

53. Mbih Jerome Tosam et al., 'Global Emerging Pathogens, Poverty and Vulnerability: An Ethical Analysis', in Godfrey Tangwa et al. (eds), *Socio-cultural Dimensions of Emerging Infectious Diseases in Africa*, Springer, 2019: 243–253, link.springer.com/chapter/10.1007/978-3-030-17474-3_18.

54. Alumdena M. Saéz et al., 'Investigation the zoonotic origin of the West African Ebola epidemic', *Embo Press*, 7 (2015): 17–23, embopress.org/doi/full/10.15252/emmm.201404792.

55. Ibid.

56. Development Initiatives, *Poverty trends: Global, regional and national*, fact sheet, 2019, devinit.org/resources/poverty-trends-global-regional-and-national/#note-Yr_3XWnJm.

57. Francisco Ferreira and Carolina Páramo-Sánchez, 'A richer array of international poverty lines', *World Bank*, 13 October 2017, blogs.worldbank.org/developmenttalk/richer-array-international-poverty-lines?CID=POV_TT_Poverty_EN_EXT.

58. Development Initiatives, *Poverty trends*.

59. The World Bank, 'COVID-19 to add as many as 150 million extreme poor by 2021', press release, 2020, www.worldbank.org/en/news/press-release/2020/10/07/covid-19-to-add-as-many-as-150-million-extreme-poor-by-2021.

60. Katherine R. Dean et al., 'Human ectoparasites and the spread of plague in Europe during the second pandemic', *PNAS*, 115/6 (2017): 1304–1309, www.pnas.org/content/115/6/1304.

61. C. J. Duncan and S. Scott, 'What caused the Black Death', *Postgraduate Medical Journal*, 81/955 (2004): 315–320, pmj.bmj.com/content/81/955/315.

62. Molly Blackall, 'Global tourism hits record highs – but who goes where on holiday?', *Guardian*, 1 July 2019, www.theguardian.com/news/2019/jul/01/global-tourism-hits-record-highs-but-who-goes-where-on-holiday.

63. Cited in Esteban Ortiz-Ospina and Diana Beltekian, *Trade and globalisation*, Our World in Data, 2018, ourworldindata.org/trade-and-globalization.

64. Ibid.

65. Kierra Box, 'The climate crisis – how international trade must change', *Friends of the Earth*, 8 February 2021, Policy.friendsoftheearth.uk/opinion/climate-crisis-how-international-trade-must-change.

66. S. M. Soto, 'Human migration and infectious diseases', *Clinical Microbiology and Infection*, 15/S1 (2009): 26–28, www.sciencedirect.com/science/article/pii/S1198743X14604080.

67. Michelle Gayer, 'Conflict and Emerging Infectious Diseases', *Emerging Infectious Diseases*, 13/11 (2007): 1625–1631, www.ncbi.nlm.nih.gov/pmc/articles/PMC3375795/.

68. Ibid.

69. Ibid

70. Mark Wheelis, 'Biological Warfare at the 1346 Siege of Caffa', *Emerging Infectious Diseases*, 8/9 (2002), wwwnc.cdc.gov/eid/article/8/9/01-0536_article.

71. Institute for Economics and Peace, *Ecological Threat Register 2020*, 2020 reliefweb.int/sites/reliefweb.int/files/resources/ETR_2020_web-1.pdf.

72. UNHCR, *UNHCR Projected Global Resettlement Needs 2021*, 2020, reliefweb.int/report/world/unhcr-projected-global-resettlement-needs-2021#:~:text=While%20in%202019%20over%2063%2C000,31%20countries%20will%20be%20met.

73. Laurie Laybourn-Langton, *Inheriting the earth? The unprecedented challenge of environmental breakdown for younger generations*, Institute of Public Policy Research, 2019, www.ippr.org/research/publications/inheriting-the-earth.

74. As per Michael Marmot et al., *The Marmot Review: 10 Years On*, Institute for Health Equity, 2020, www.instituteofhealthequity.org/resources-reports/marmot-review-10-years-on.

75. HM Government, *Contained and controlled: The UK's 20-year vision for antimicrobial resistance*, 2019, assets.publishing.service.gov.uk/government/uploads/system/uploads/attachment_data/file/773065/uk-20-year-vision-for-antimicrobial-resistance.pdf.

76. Ibid.

77. Nick Allen, 'Humans could live to 100, say scientists', *The Telegraph*, 27 May 2021, www.telegraph.co.uk/news/2021/05/27/humans-could-live-150-say-scientists/.

78. Kyree Leary, 'Ageing expert: The first person to live to 1,000 has already been born', *Futurism*, 1 December 2017, futurism.com/aging-expert-person-1000-born; Rob Waugh, 'The first immortals have already been born, Cambridge scientist claims', *Metro*, 14 April 2015, metro.co.uk/2015/04/14/

the-first-immortals-have-already-been-born-cambridge-scientist-claims-5149788/.

79. Laurie Laybourn-Langton et al., *Inheriting the earth?*, Institute for Public Policy Research, September 2019, www.ippr.org/files/2019-11/inheriting-the-earth-july19.pdf.

80. See Stian Westlake, *The end of the Treasury: Breaking up the UK's finance ministry*, Nesta, 3 September 2014, www.nesta.org.uk/report/the-end-of-the-treasury-breaking-up-the-uks-finance-ministry/.

81. For example, the Treasury Select Committee generated very unfavourable headlines for David Cameron, over his involvement in Lobbying for Greensill Capital to be given government contracts. Treasury Select Committee, 'Treasury Committee reports on 'lessons from Greensill Capital'', 2021, https://committees.parliament.uk/committee/158/treasury-committee/news/156684/treasury-committee-reports-on-lessons-from-greensill-capital/.

82. RAN, *The dirty dozen*, 2020, www.ran.org/bankingonclimatechaos 2021/#data-panel.

83. Facing Finance, *Dirty profits 7*, 2019, www.facing-finance.org/files/2019/05/ff_dp7_ONLINE_v02.pdf.

84. Banks have long funded these activities. See also: War on Want, *Deadly investments*, 2017, waronwant.org/sites/default/files/Final%20Web%20version%20Deadly%20Investments.pdf.

85. Green New Deal Group, *A Green New Deal*, 2008, https://neweconomics.org/uploads/files/8f737ea195fe56db2f_xbm6ihwb1.pdf.

86. Luke Murphy et al., *Fairness and opportunity*, Institute of Public Policy Research, 2021, Ippr.org/research/publications/fairness-and-opportunity.

87. OECD, *Main science and technology indicators*, dataset, 2021, data.oecd.org/rd/gross-domestic-spending-on-r-d.htm.

88. Shreya Nanda and Chris Thomas, *The science-based economy: The role of health research*, Institute of Public Policy Research, 2020, www.ippr.org/files/2020-07/1594310646_the-science-based-economy-july20.pdf.

89. The exception to this are infectious diseases, where there is a very good case for disproportionate investment on a humanitarian basis.

90. Overall impact in this case means 'Quality-Adjusted Life Years' – a measure that accounts both for quality and length of life.

91. Shreya Nanda and Chris Thomas, *The science-based economy*.

92. Jon Sussex et al., 'Quantifying the economic impact of government and charity funding of medical research on private research and development funding in the United Kingdom', *BMC*, 14/32 (2016), bmcmedicine.biomedcentral.com/articles/10.1186/s12916-016-0564-z

93. For more on the worth of public and charity spending on medical research see King's College London, RAND Europe, Brunel University London, *Medical research: What's it worth?*, research briefing, 2018, acmedsci.ac.uk/file-download/54792223.

CHAPTER 6

1. Douglas Holtz-Eakin et al., *The Green New Deal: Scope, scale and implications*, American Action Forum, 2019, www.americanactionforum. org/research/the-green-new-deal-scope-scale-and-implications/.
2. Lord Ara Darzi et al., *Better health and care for all*, Institute for Public Policy Research, 2018, www.ippr.org/research/publications/ better-health-and-care-for-all.
3. Chris Thomas, *Resilient health and care*, Institute of Public Policy Research, 2020, ippr.org/research/publications/resilient-health-and-care. This estimate uses latest estimates available, meaning it does not account for how similar nations healthcare spending will settle following the pandemic.
4. Chris Thomas et al., *The innovation lottery: Upgrading the spread of innovation in the NHS*, Institute of Public Policy Research, 2020, www.ippr. org/research/publications/the-innovation-lottery.
5. As per Chris Thomas, *Resilient health and care*.
6. As costed by Labour Party, *Care for carers*, 2020, labour.org.uk/wp-content/ uploads/2020/06/CFCfinal-v2.pdf.
7. As concluded by Luke Raikes et al., *Divided and connected: Regional inequalities in the north, the UK and the developed world – State of the North 2019*, Institute of Public Policy Research North, 2019, www.ippr.org/ research/publications/state-of-the-north-2019.
8. Dean Hochlaf and Chris Thomas, *The whole society approach*, Institute of Public Policy Research, 2020, www.ippr.org/research/publications/ the-whole-society-approach.
9. UCL Institute for Global Prosperity, *Social prosperity for the future: A proposal for Universal Basic Services*, 2017, www.ucl.ac.uk/bartlett/igp/ sites/bartlett/files/universal_basic_services_-_the_institute_for_global_ prosperity_.pdf.
10. Department for Education, *Consolidated annual report and accounts*, HM Government, 2020, https://assets.publishing.service.gov.uk/government/ uploads/system/uploads/attachment_data/file/932898/DfE_consolidated_ annual_report_and_accounts_2019_to_2020__web_version_.pdf.
11. Labour for UBS, *Universal Basic Services manifesto*, 2020, labourforubs.files. wordpress.com/2020/09/labourforubs-policy-consultation-document.pdf.
12. Patel et al., *The state of health and care*.
13. Alfie Stirling and Joe Dromey, *Uncapped potential*, Institute of Public Policy Research, 2017, www.ippr.org/files/2017-11/uncapped-potential-november2017.pdf; London Economics, *The net exchequer impact of increasing pay for agenda for change staff*, 2021, londoneconomics.co.uk/ blog/publication/the-net-exchequer-impact-of-increasing-pay-for-agenda-for-change-staff/.
14. OECD, *Environmental taxation*, data, 2020, www.oecd.org/env/tools-evaluation/environmentaltaxation.htm.
15. National Food Strategy, *The plan*, 2021, www.nationalfoodstrategy.org/.
16. Westminster could not introduce public health net zero across all four nations, as powers to this end are devolved.

17. Patel et al., *State of Health and Care.*
18. Chris Thomas, *Community first social care.*
19. Harry Quilter-Pinner, *Social care: Free at the point of need,* Institute of Public Policy Research, 2019, www.ippr.org/files/2019-05/social-care-free-at-the-point-of-need-may-19.pdf.
20. I.e., the £5 billion a year should not count towards government targets on R&D reaching certain per centages of UK GDP.
21. Harry Quilter-Pinner and Dean Hochlaf, *Austerity: There is an alternative and the UK can afford to deliver it,* Institute of Public Policy Research, 2019, www.ippr.org/blog/austerity-there-is-an-alternative-and-the-uk-can-afford-to-deliver-it.
22. Alfie Stirling and Sarah Arnold, 'Austerity by stealth?', *New Economics Foundation,* 17 September 2018, neweconomics.org/2018/09/austerity-by-stealth.
23. Carsten Jung et al., *Boost it like Biden,* Institute of Public Policy Research, 2021, www.ippr.org/research/publications/boost-it-like-biden.
24. Often thought to require its own £50–£100 billion investment programme – as per Tax Research UK, *Funding the UK Green New Deal,* 2019, www.taxresearch.org.uk/Blog/2019/09/16/funding-the-uk-green-new-deal/, or the commitment of £100 billion investment in the 2019 Green Party manifesto or Green New Deal Group, *A national plan for the UK,* 2013, greennewdealgroup.org/wp-content/uploads/2013/09/Green-New-Deal-5th-Anniversary.pdf.
25. Ibid.
26. I.e., Chris Thomas, *The 'make do and mend' health service: Solving the NHS's capital crisis,* Institute of Public Policy Research, 2019, www.ippr.org/files/2019-09/1568215446_the-make-do-and-mend-health-service-summary.pdf.
27. British Medical Association, *Workload undermines PCNs, finds survey,* 2020, www.bma.org.uk/news-and-opinion/workload-undermines-pcns-finds-survey.
28. Nicola Merrifield, 'GPs working average 11-hour day, major survey finds', *Pulse Today,* 1 April 2021, www.pulsetoday.co.uk/news/workload/gps-working-average-11-hour-day-major-survey-reveals/.
29. Chris Thomas and Harry Quilter-Pinner, *Realising the neighbourhood NHS,* Institute of Public Policy Research, 2020, www.ippr.org/research/publications/realising-the-neighbourhood-nhs.
30. NHS Digital, *General practice workforce,* data collection, 2019, digital.nhs.uk/data-and-information/publications/statistical/general-and-personal-medical-services.
31. Though not unheard off. It was called for by the then Labour MP and GP Paul Williams in 2019. Paul Williams, 'As a doctor, I say it's time to nationalise GP surgeries', *Guardian,* 8 May 2019, www.theguardian.com/commentisfree/2019/may/08/gp-nationalise-surgeries-profit-patients-nhs.
32. Probably because their policy is designed by councils of senior doctors who benefit from that status quo.

33. Recreated from Chris Thomas et al., *Levelling-up health for prosperity*, Institute of Public Policy Research/IPPR North, 2020, www.ippr.org/research/publications/levelling-up-health-for-prosperity; Data from Public Health England, *Public health profiles*, data, 2020, fingertips.phe.org.uk/.

34. Chris Thomas et al., *Levelling-up health for prosperity*.

35. The King's Fund, *A Citizen-led approach to health and care: lessons from the Wigan Deal*, 2019, www.kingsfund.org.uk/sites/default/files/2019-06/A_citizen-led_approach_to_health_and_care_lessons_from_the_Wigan_Deal_summary.pdf.

36. Ibid.

37. As per Centre for Public Impact, *The Wigan deal*, 2020, www.centreforpublicimpact.org/case-study/the-wigan-deal.

38. Preston City Council, CLES, *How we built community wealth in Preston*, 2019, www.preston.gov.uk/media/1792/How-we-built-community-wealth-in-Preston/pdf/CLES_Preston_Document_WEB_AW.pdf?m=636994067328930000.

39. Paul Dennett, 'Sensible socialism: The Salford Model', *Tribune*, 19 January 2021, tribunemag.co.uk/2021/01/sensible-socialism-the-salford-model.

40. Ipsos Mori, 'Britains are most likely to think their health care system is overstretched', press release, 1 December 2020, www.ipsos.com/ipsos-mori/en-uk/britons-are-most-likely-think-their-healthcare-system-overstretched.

41. Health Foundation, *What does the public think about NHS and Social Care Services?*, 2017, www.health.org.uk/publications/reports/what-does-the-public-think-about-nhs-and-social-care-services.

EPILOGUE

1. See Richard Sloggett, 'Why both sides want to play political football with the NHS', *Times Red Box*, 19 November 2019, www.thetimes.co.uk/article/why-both-sides-want-to-play-political-football-with-the-nhs-2m6xxjq9d.

2. Ipsos Mori, *Issues Index December 2020*, 2020, www.ipsos.com/sites/default/files/ct/news/documents/2020-01/issues_index_december2019_v1_public.pdf; Ipsos Mori, *Issues index archives*, dataset, www.ipsos.com/ipsos-mori/en-uk/issues-index-2007-onwards; Ipsos Mori, *Best party on key issues: Health care*, www.ipsos.com/ipsos-mori/en-uk/best-party-key-issues-health-care.

3. 1992 has the bearings of a Labour election victory, both in health and beyond. This is true for other issues too – the Conservatives won despite a long period in governance, rising unemployment rates, a long recession, high interest rates and house price collapse. In this case, Labour faced a perfect storm of structural problems – from unpopular leadership, to the media environment, to socio-demographic change – that help explain this outlier.

4. Indicatively, see Tom Harwood, 'Labour's NHS Scaremongering is Based on Shameless Lies', *Free Market Conservatives*, 2019, freemarketconservatives. org/labours-nhs-scaremongering-is-based-on-shameless-lies/.
5. Jack Peat, 'Two in five healthcare workers voted conservative in local elections', *The London Economic*, 2021, www.thelondoneconomic.com/ politics/two-in-five-healthcare-workers-voted-conservative-in-local-elections-268479/.

Index

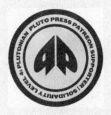

Thanks to our Patreon subscriber:

Ciaran Kane

Who has shown generosity and comradeship in support of our publishing.

Check out the other perks you get by subscribing to our Patreon – visit patreon.com/plutopress. Subscriptions start from £3 a month.

The Pluto Press Newsletter

Hello friend of Pluto!

Want to stay on top of the best radical books
we publish?

Then sign up to be the first to hear about our
new books, as well as special events,
podcasts and videos.

You'll also get 50% off your first order with us
when you sign up.

Come and join us!

Go to bit.ly/PlutoNewsletter

Printed and bound by CPI Group (UK) Ltd, Croydon, CR0 4YY

16/07/2023

03236607-0001